Timing and the Times

Chronicity in the American Practice of Oriental Medicine

by

Bob Flaws
Charles Chace
Michael Helme

Blue Poppy Press

Published by:

BLUE POPPY PRESS
2140 Pine St.
Boulder, CO 80302

First Edition
May 1986

ISBN 0-936185-04-X

Other Books by Bob Flaws:

PATH OF PREGNANCY

PRINCE WEN HUI'S COOK (with Honora Lee Wolfe)

TIEH TA KE (formerly titled HIT MEDICINE)

TURTLE TAIL & OTHER TENDER MERCIES

BLUE POPPY QIGONG

My son, you should not belittle (the practice of medicine) because it is apparently but a matter of herbs and trees. You should endeavor to penetrate to the realm where Essence (JING) and Spirit (SHEN) are joined and proceed to the border regions where the dark meets the mysterious. Once you understand the beginning and the end of all processes and once you have grasped the origin and consequences of a result, it can be said that you have accomplished something in the field (of medicine). You certainly must take the greatest pains!

(From Chang Chieh-pin's CHANG SHIH CHING YO CHUAN SHU, circa 1624 CE, based on a translation by Paul Unschuld appearing in MEDICAL ETHICS IN IMPERIAL CHINA, UC PRESS, CA 1979)

TABLE OF CONTENTS

INTRODUCTION

Since the publication of ESSENTIALS OF CHINESE ACUPUNCTURE and ACUPUNCTURE: A COMPREHENSIVE TEXT, the basic rudiments of Chinese medicine have been made available to westerners. These two texts are the foundation of the curricula of most American acupuncture schools and are the criteria for facticity on American licensure exams. Since they are beginners' texts they are limited in scope. However, what is not also commonly appreciated is that they present a particular version of Chinese medicine in the guise of a single orthodoxy. Ted Kaptchuk's THE WEB THAT HAS NO WEAVER similarly presents this same style to both lay and professional readers as if it were the definitive one. Likewise this is the style presented by Manfred Porkert in ESSENTIALS OF CHINESE DIAGNOSIS. This style is known as Traditional Chinese Medicine or TCM and is the state-approved one in the People's Republic of China. That this is a style of Chinese medicine has been recognized by Ted Kaptchuk in a book review published in the JOURNAL OF CHINESE MEDICINE where he says, "Traditional Chinese Medicine is not necessarily equivalent to all the different traditional healing methods in China, even if they share such words as qi."[1] Dr. Kaptchuk in an earlier issue of the same publication has stated that, "The treatments that are now being used in China I think come from the 1930's with a modification in the last ten years..."[2]

The practice of Chinese medicine by and for non-Asians is a recent phenomenon here in the US. It is hardly more than ten years old. As in any "new" profession, in the beginning, information on Chinese medicine was scant, incomplete, and often inaccurate. With the publication of ESSENTIALS, COMPREHENSIVE, and WEB, a second phase has been completed, i.e. the establishment of a legitimate foundation for the clinical study and practice of Chinese medicine in America. During this phase practitioners have learned or are learning the rudiments of our art at an entry level. However, in my opinion, the next phase requires two separate endeavors. The first is the expansion of the number of primary source texts made available in English. The second is the creation of a western literature addressing the peculiar health needs of this time and place.

In order to get a fuller, more mature, and historically accurate view of the depth and breadth of Chinese medicine we need access to a much larger cross-section of Chinese medical literature, both classical and contemporary. Chinese medical literature spans two millenia and is not homogeneous. Many different theories and trends have come and gone over the centuries and there are written records of these. Chinese medical theories and techniques are the product of social, cultural, philosophical, and historical factors. It is necessary to be aware of these factors in assessing the value or relevancy of any particular theory or technique.

For instance, today's TCM style of Chinese medicine seems to me to have been heavily influenced by the YEN LI or HAN XUE PAI school of Chinese philosophy of the Qing dynasty. This school was a reaction against Neoconfuscianism. Neoconfuscianist philosophy was based largely on the mystical insights of Buddhism and Taoism. Neoconfuscianism was the philosophical basis which allowed for the great flowering of classical Chinese medicine in the Song, Jin, Yuan, and Ming dynasties. The YEN LI philosophers, on the other hand, such as Wang Fu-chi, Li Kung, and Tai Chen, embraced a form of outright materialism and rejected meditation and introspection as ways to intuit the principles of an Idealist reality. These philosophers stripped the spiritual implications from such words as JING, QI, and SHEN. Consciousness became merely epiphenomenal and human life was denuded of its mystical teleological purpose. This materialist philosophy set the stage for the Chinese enthusiasm for western science and their adoption of such a materialistic, humanistic social philosophy as Communism. This HAN XUE PAI philosophical movement catalyzed renewed interest in Han dynasty medicine as embodied in the SHAN HAN LUN and was directly responsible for the numerous commentaries written on that classic in the eighteenth and nineteenth centuries. Happily, not all Chinese philosophers and physicians have accepted this YEN LI philosophy. However, without knowing about the historical debate between Neoconfuscianist and YEN LI philosophy, one cannot recognize clearly and descriminate between the various styles of contemporary Chinese medicine based on these respective points of view.

This is basic scholarship. If we are to take advantage of Chinese medicine's unique and extensive literature, we must develop descrimination based on knowing who said what when. At an earlier stage in our western interest in Chinese medicine, writers could get away with saying that the Chinese believe this or that without documentation. This is akin to saying that Americans play basketball. Well, some Americans do, but I am an American and I don't. The uncritical acceptance of such generalizations typifies the naiveté characteristic of neophytes. Now, as we and our profession emerge from our infancy in the West, we need to develop a connoisseurship commensurate with maturity.

This type of scholarship largely represents a conscious turning back to the past to consolidate our foundation in the present. It is not a worshipping of some bygone era with nostalgic reverence. It is simply the conscious acknowledgement of where we are being a function of where we have come from. And it is only by knowing where we have come from and therefore where we are that we can chart the course of where we are going. The translations excerpted from the ZHEN JIU DA CHENG and the life's works of Jin Zi-jiu and Wang Le-ting are offered below in this spirit. They are building blocks with which to create our own conceptual edifice. The ZHEN JIU DA CHENG is one of, if not the most widely respected Chinese classics on the practice of acupuncture and moxabustion. It is the summation of the majority of previous Chinese theory and clinical experience on this subject up to the Ming dynasty. The writings of Jin Zi-jiu and Wang Le-ting, on the other hand, exemplify how recent Old Masters have worked creatively within the conceptual framework of Chinese medicine. I believe they convey a sense of an individual's experience and point of view. For me their writings de-emphasize that there is a monolithic orthodoxy in this art. Once we as practitioners are knowledgable enough to say that this doctor living at this time and in this place said this and that, we then gain a conceptual space within which we can maneuver. Whereas, saying Chinese medicine says this or that creates the impression of solidity which is not conducive to creativity. Rather it fosters the impression of a <u>fait accompli</u>.

Having shorn up our conceptual foundation by scholarship into our roots, it seems to me that we, as western practitioners, must also endeavor to think creatively with the concepts of Chinese medicine in a way that is relevant to our time and place. So far we have been so busy learning to copy how the Chinese have used these concepts that few of us had had the time to think about their larger philosophical implications in terms of our own experience. However, for me the spirit of Chinese medicine is the moment by moment assessment of the Qi at a given time and place which is by nature unique. Therefore what worked in China two thousand years ago may not work here in twentieth century America. Whether any particular theory or technique is relevant to our situation will depend on years, if not generations, of clinical experience and research. Yet, until we begin to consciously discuss and relate Chinese theory and practice to our present situation, we will only be imitating someone else's form.

The principles of Chinese medicine are concepts, ideas -- abstractions. As such they transcend culture and even time. The employment of these principles as treatment in the human realm, however, is by necessity a function of time and place and therefore must take these factors into conscious account. In Chinese, the term ZHI YI means "treatment compatibility". There are three categories of changing circumstances which must be taken into account when erecting a treatment plan which is situationally appropriate. These are time, place, and the idiosyncracies of the individual.[3] On a prosaic level this means adjusting a treatment because of weather, the phase of the moon, the season of the year, etc. However, on a larger level, it means that the entirety of Chinese medical theory and practice must be adjusted to meet the historical needs of any patient population. The principles of Chinese medicine are based on ontological and cosmological speculation. They are a species of philosophy. In fact, as discussed above, there are more than one style of Chinese medicine based on more than one philosophical point of view. It seems to me that western practitioners must begin to think about these principles' philosophical implications in a more profound and ultimately relevant way. Although we need more case histories and articles on the differentiation of syndromes to complete the cross-referencing of western named diseases with their equivalent Chinese patterns of disharmony, we also need a higher type of philosophical discussion to continuely expand and quicken the living spirit of our art.

Harris Coulter in DIVIDED LEGACY: A HISTORY OF THE SCHISM IN MEDICAL THOUGHT divides all medical thought into two broad categories. That which is based on metaphysical principles he calls Rational. That which is based on individual experience he call Empirical.[4] Based on Coulter's dichotomy, the YEN LI influenced practitioners are the Emprirics of Oriental medicine. In Japan exponents of the HAN XUE PAI, such as Nagoya Geni, Goto Gonzan, Kagawa Shuan, and Yoshimasu Tode, echoed the same arguments of contemporaneous Empirics in Europe such as Paracelsus, Von Helmont, and Hahnemann.[5] Neoconfuscian-influenced practitioners are the Chinese counterparts of western Galenic or Rationalist schools, although this dichotomy is not as pronounced in the history of Chinese medicine as it is in the western. "Not that every practitioner of medicine falls exclusively into one or the other tradition. The run-of-the-mill physician concerns himself essentially with the technical problem of applying given therapeutic rules to his patient's needs. He does not question the postulates and assumptions behind the rules he has learned because he is not aware of them. His practice is an eclectic and inconsistent mixture of the two bodies of doctrine. But the greatest thinkers fall on one or the other end of this spectrum of thought. They are great precisely because they have examined the underlying assumptions and on them have erected coherent bodies of doctrine."[6] Although the pendular swing from Empiric to Rationalist perspectives in medicine seems to be perpetual, and even natural, still the time is ripe for renewed discussion of the fundamental existential and philosophical implications of the theories underlying various styles of Chinese medicine. It is only from out of an environment of intellectual ferment that great thought can arise.

To date only a very few practitioners of Oriental medicine writing for westerners have entered upon such philosophical discussion. Professor Worsley in England has developed a style of acupuncture based on a non-TCM interpretation of Five Element theory and an almost Freudian theory of the cause of disease which has caused a great deal of discussion in the international acupuncture community. His techniques as practiced by himself and his many students have successfully treated, it would seem, thousands of western patients. Unfortunately the paucity of scholarship employed by himself and his students in their writings has led many adherents of other styles to dismiss this style as bogus. This is a great shame since Prof. Worsley's style and theory raise many questions germaine to the practice of acupuncture on twentieth century western patients. Macrobiotic practitioners, such as Ohsawa, Kushi, and Muramoto, have likewise discussed many important sociological, philosophical, and cosmological issues in their writings. Once again, however, their poor documentation and scholarship and their idiosyncratic and critically unexplained use of such seminal terms as Yin and Yang have obscured their potential relevance for adherents of other styles of Oriental healing. It is too easy to dismiss their theories as unfounded and therefore to overlook the important issues they raise. Ted Kaptchuk, on the other hand, is one of the only writers on Oriental medicine who has both supported his writings with impeccable and extensive scholarship and examined Chinese medicine's relevance for westerners on a philosophical level. Although I do not always agree with Dr. Kaptchuk's opinions and conclusions, I applaud the level of intelligence exhibited in his work and his attempt at creating a meaningful dialogue.

Chinese medicine is only one therapeutic option available to late twentieth century Americans. Our culture and indeed our entire planet are facing a crisis on both physical and spiritual levels. If prospective patients are to recognize the special character and qualities of our vision of health and treatment we must address ourselves as practitioners of Chinese medicine to the larger existential issues with which we are all faced. If we truly believe Chinese medicine's vision of microcosmic/macrocosmic unity, then the zeitgeist must be assessed and taken into account in the treatment of our patients.

This is not to say that we should rush out to immediately create an American version of Chinese medicine. Such will evolve naturally and organically over several generations just as Korean, Vietnamese, and Japanese versions have evolved in their countries. An American version will not be the sole creation of a single individual. The present is part of a continuum between past and future. Rigid conservatism is dead and unresponsive. It is limited by what was. But wholesale abandonment of tradition cuts one's roots and foundation. Substantial change is always organic. It is seldom consciously planned by one or even a group of individuals. What is necessary now is to raise the questions and issues which our medicine must struggle to address as it takes root in our environment. It is the raising of these questions and the discussion and contemplation of these issues which are important at this time. Only history will tell if any of the answers we might also propose stand the test of time. That does not matter. What matters is that, in all our discussions of tongue and pulse and signs and symptoms, we also probe the logical, ontological, epistemological, ethical, and existential implications of our practice.

The following essays all have to do with some aspect of timing or the times in which we live in the practice of Oriental medicine. As a member of a Buddhist tradition of medicine, my philosophic point of view is closer to the Neoconfuscianist perspective than the YEN LI influenced TCM one. It is my belief that greater attention to Buddhist, Taoist, and Neoconfuscian theories and styles of Oriental medicine is the necessary corrective for the over-secularization and materialization of contemporary medical practice, both eastern and western. Since disease is a species of suffering, I believe it ultimately requires a spiritual cure and that any medicine which does not acknowledge and address that necessity cannot cure disease at its root and is therefore liable to cause further problems. Not all readers are likely to agree with this belief, but, if the following essays catalyze discussion of these issues amongst American practitioners of Oriental medicine, they will have served their purpose.

The excerpts from the ZHEN JIU DA CHENG published below have been translated by Charles Chace. Those from JIN ZHEN WANG LE-TING and JIN ZI-JIU ZHUAN JI were translated by Michael Helme. We would like to thank Kiko Matsumoto for her inspiration and encouragement in researching various passages from the ZHEN JIU DA CHANG and MING TANG MOXA CLASSIC. Drs. Huang Pao-chin and Zhou Ming-ying also graciously assisted in elucidating some difficult passages.

Bob Flaws
Feb. 20, 1986
Boulder, CO

ENDNOTES

1 Kaptchuk, Ted, "Another Look at Qi: A Book Review of ENCOUNTERS WITH QI: EXPLORING CHINESE MEDICINE by David Eisenberg", JOURNAL OF CHINESE MEDICINE, UK, #19, Sept. 1985, p. 32

2 Kaptchuk, Ted, "Acupuncture in the West -- a discussion between Ted Kaptchuk, Giovanni Maciocia, Felicity Moir, and Peter Deadman", JOURNAL OF CHINESE MEDICINE, UK, #17, Jan. 1985, p. 26

3 Liu Yan-mau, CHINESE MEDICAL TERMINOLOGY, The Commercial Press Ltd., HK, date ?, p. 130

4 Coulter, Harris L., DIVIDED LEGACY: A HISTORY OF THE SCHISM IN MEDICAL THOUGHT, Weehawken Books, Wash. DC, 1975, p. xiii

5 Otsuka, Yasuo, "Chinese Traditional Medicine in Japan", ASIAN MEDICAL SYSTEMS, ed. by Charles Leslie, U of CA Press, Berkeley, 1976, p. 328-330

6 Coulter, op. cit., p. xiii

THE TALE OF THE RED-TIPPED TONGUE

Chinese & Tibetan Medical Perspectives on Neurasthenia

One day I was examining a patient whose major complaint was recurring and incapacitating knee pain. He was in his early thirties. His knees had been painful off and on for three years. They seemed to be worse in the winter, the pain was fixed in location, and it was relieved somewhat by soaking in warm water. The man worked nights as a waiter and he had had a long history of marijuana abuse. I did not consider his pulse or tongue remarkable. Since this seemed to be a BI or Obstruction syndrome of the meridians, I did not pay much attention to either. Since the patient lived at some distance and acupuncture was therefore not feasible, I began writing a Chinese herbal prescription for Cold BI of the lower extremities.

Just as I had finished composing the formula, Zhou Ming-ying, a young Chinese doctor from Shangahi studying in Boulder, stopped by to visit my wife. Considering this a fortuitous opportunity for the patient to have my diagnosis and prescription checked by another, and better trained, practitioner of Chinese medicine, I asked Dr. Zhou to look at my formula and give her opinion. She asked the patient one or two questions about the nature and location of his pain. Then she asked to see his tongue. She took me to one side and told me I had better look at the tongue again, that my formula was too Hot for this patient.

I took Dr. Zhou's advice and examined the tongue again. The tongue was a bit fluted at its lower edge, was normally furred, but did have a pronounced red tip. This was the Heat that Dr. Zhou was referring to. Following Dr. Zhou's recommendation, I removed the Radix Aconite from the formula and instead added more Blood and Yin tonics such as Radix Paeonia alba and Tang Kuei. Within less than a week the patient reported back that his knee pain was much improved and has not bothered now for over a year.

I was very grateful to Dr. Zhou for pointing out my oversight. Over the next several weeks my mind kept returning to this patient and his red-tipped tongue. I realized that I am so used to seeing red-tipped tongues that I had gotten into the habit of discounting them as the "standard" red-tipped tongue. It was as if a red-tipped tongue had become a expected norm in my patient population. Dr. Zhou's correction of my failure to take this patient's red-tipped tongue into proper account led me to consider the meanings and implications of this commonly encountered diagnostic sign.

I practice in Boulder, Colorado. Boulder is a university city known for its liberal environment with a sophisticated lifestyle. The city abounds with restaurants, cafes, movies, and every other manner of entertainment, both legal and illegal. In the early seventies it was a bastion of radical hippiedom. Now it is a capital of yuppiedom. The majority of my patients are in their late twenties to late thirties. The majority of my practice is devoted to gynecological disorders, although I do conduct a general practice, treating everything from pediatric problems to traumatic injuries to systemic diseases such as MS and Lupus. However, within my main patient population of persons between the ages of twenty and forty, I would estimate that a full 90% exhibit the red-tipped tongue.

According to Traditional Chinese Medicine, what does a red-tipped tongue indicate? To answer that question we must first examine the place of inspection of the tongue within the context of the traditional Four Methods of diagnosis. Inspection of the tongue is perhaps one of the most important inspections in contemporary Chinese medicine. In the differentiation of syndromes it accounts for one third of the diagnosis, the other two thirds being comprised of pulse palpation and signs and symptoms, the symptoms being primarily elicited by interrogation or questioning.

Inspection of the tongue is perhaps the clearest diagnostic method for determining the condition of the patient, symptoms often being confusing and the pulse being obscure due to its subtlety. Looking at the tongue is looking at the inside of the body itself. In particular, the tongue is the most reliable indicator of the presence or absence of Heat in the body, while the pulse is a more accurate measure of Excess or Deficiency. Determining whether a patient is a Hot or Cold conformation is one of the four dichotomies traditionally known as the Eight Principles. This determination is absolutely essential for correct treatment since the heteropathic logic of Chinese medicine demands that pathologic Heat be cooled, while pathologic Cold should be warmed.

When examining the tongue there are two basic divisions: the assessment of the tongue proper or the "meat" and the assessment of the coating or "fur". In assessing the meat, color is the major indicator of the presence or absence of Heat in the patient, a redder than normal tongue indicating Heat and a paler tongue the absence of Heat, or Cold. Abnormal coloration of the tongue may be generalized but it often is restricted to a specific or limited area. In Chinese tongue diagnosis, different areas of the tongue are believed to correspond to particular internal organs. In general, we can say that the rear third of the tongue corresponds to the Lower Burner, the middle third to the Middle Burner, and the apical third to the Upper Burner. Within this scheme, the tip itself corresponds to the Heart. Therefore a red tip of the tongue indicates a pathologic accumulation of Heat in the Upper Burner in general and in the Heart in particular.

This belief is unanimously accepted in all Chinese diagnostic literature with which I am familiar. The PIEN SHE CHIH NAN states: "Only the tongue apex is red and is beginning to develop prickles as the result of over-thriving fire in the heart."[1] The CHUNG I SHE CHEN states: "The tongue color in most cases must be light (in) color with some being bright red which depends on the location of the color ... Red on the apex and sides is evidence that the heart and liver are feverish."[2] Yang Chih-yi notes in his discussion of tongue diagnosis that "(if) only the apex of the tongue appears dark red, it indicates a thriving heart fire."[3] Pao Tien-pai says, "If only the tongue apex developes prickles, it is called 'heart fire flare-up'."[4] ACUPUNCTURE: A COMPREHENSIVE TEXT[5] says, "Red eruptions on the tip or edges of the tongue indicate intense Heat." It goes on to say that, "In conditions of Excessive Heat the entire tongue is red, whereas with Deficient Heat only the tip is so colored."[6]

These Chinese sources are echoed by western exponents of Traditional Chinese Medicine as well. Manfred Porkert states that, "If the scarlet colouring is restricted to the tip of the tongue, we may conclude that 'glare' (Heat) is present in the o. cardialis (i.e. the Heart)."[7] And finally, Ted Kaptchuk writes that, "Red eruptions, pimples, or thornlike protrusions on the tongue, redder than the occasional raised papillae of the normal tongue, are usually signs of Heat or Congealed Blood ... These signs often occur on only certain portions of the tongue ... For such cases particular areas of the tongue are said to correspond to particular Organs."[8]

Not only are the overwhelming majority of writers agreed that a red tongue tip signifies pathologic Heat in the Heart, but the Chinese medical tradition from the time of the NEI JING is unanimous in asserting that the tongue has special relationship with the Heart. Ted Kaptchuk, quoting from the SU WEN, expresses this realationship succinctly: "'The Heart opens into the tongue.' ... The tradition also says that 'the tongue is the sprout of the Heart.' the tongue is closely realated to the Heart Qi and Heart Blood. This means that if disharmonies occur in the Heart, they are sometimes discernible in the tongue."[9]

So, a red-tipped tongue indicates Heat accumulating within the Heart. This Heat is a local Excess since it is not supposed to be there. However, when seen systemically, this Heat is not a true Excess but rather a Deficiency Heat. The reader must be careful to note that this is not a Deficiency <u>of</u> Heat but rather Heat due to a Deficiency. The energy which is Deficient which allows for the production of this Heat is the True Yin. The root of this True Yin is the kidney Yin or Kidney Water. It is the diminishment of this Yin which allows this Heat to rise up into the Heart.

In my experience, tongue diagnosis usually confirms this scenario of Heat evaporating the Yin, especially of the Kidneys, which then burns out of control and rises to the Heart. What I have noted in my practice is the common combination of a red-tipped tongue with a tender appearance of the meat, indentations of the teeth along the formward edges, a relatively smooth surface texture with unobtrusive papillae except at the tip, and a tendency to quiver upon presentation. Although scalloping on the lateral edges of the tongue usually indicates a Damp Spleen, indentations on the tip signify Kidney Deficiency. The fact there are relatively few obtrusive papillae giving the surface a smoother than normal texture indicates the poor interrelationship between the Upper and Lower Burners and therefore a Deficiency of Righteous Qi. Ma Chien-chung states that, "The ancients considered a tongue surface with pliable prickles to be the result of the pulmonary chi being evaporated by a true renal fire. This is the normal, (whereas) few or no pliable prickles indicates the normal chi is weak."[10] And finally, as Porkert says, "A quivering tongue indicates exhaustion or ventus (Wind) of the o. hepaticus (i.e. Liver). If a quivering tongue is red, and if the speech is impeded, there is energetic deficiency in the cardinal (Heart) and lienal (Spleen) orbs."[11]

This Heat, which is both the result of pathologic changes in the organism and the cause of further problems, will have a tendency to do several things. First it will disturb the SHEN or Spirit. The LING SHU states, "The Heart stores the Shen."[12] As Kaptchuk says, "When the Heart's Blood and Qi are harmonious, Shen is nourished, and the individual responds appropriately to the environment. When the Shen-storing of the Heart is impaired, the individual may show symptoms associated with the Shen, such as insomnia, excessive dreaming, or forgetfulness. More serious disorders of this type are hysteria, irrational behavior, insanity, and delirium."[13]

Secondly, this Heat will exhaust both the Heart Yin and the Heart Qi. Although the Fire in the Heart is a species of local Excess, the Heart itself becomes Deficient. Since it is the Heart Qi and Yin (including the Blood) which "secure" and "nourish" the SHEN, the SHEN will become even more disturbed.

And third, as the Heart becomes weakened it will have repercussions on the health of the other organs in ways predictable according to the theories of Chinese medicine. According to the Creation Cycle of Five Phase Theory, the Liver is the Mother of the Heart. If the Heart becomes Deficient, the Liver will try to make up this deficit from its own Righteous Qi. In this case, it is specifically the Yin which is Deficient and so the Flaring of Fire in the Heart will tend to exhaust the Liver Yin as well. This then causes the Liver to become overheated which is a troublesome complication since in most cases the Liver is the source of the Evil Heat in the first place. Symptoms associated with Flaring of Liver Fire area bitter taste in the mouth, headaches, insomnia, and irritability.

Again according to the Creation Cycle, the Kidney will attempt to replenish the Deficiency of the Liver. As the Kidney Yin is sucked up into the Liver and Heart, it leaves the Kidney Water Deficient. It is the Kidney Water which, however, is meant to keep Heart Fire in check according to the so-called Control Cycle. If the Kidney Water becomes too weak to exercise sufficient control over Heart Fire, the Fire in the Heart will burn out of control, evaporating the Yin drafted up through the Liver and the whole process will gain a hard-to-stop momentum. the relationship between Kidney Water and Heart Fire symbolizes the primal relationship between Yin and Yang or Earth and Heaven within the human microcosm. Since disease at root is defined as a loss of balance or equilibrium between Yin and Yang in Chinese medicine, this particular imbalance between the Kidney and Heart is an ominous one.

The source of the Heart's True or Righteous Fire is the Kidney Yang or MING MEN HUO. As the Kidney Yin is depleted, the Kidney Fire will flare. This Heat will exacerbate all pathologic manifestations of Ministerial Fire in the body, whether in the Liver, Gallbladder, or Stomach and will add fuel to the

Heart Fire since Heat inevitably rises. If Kidney Yin and Yang come so far out of balance so as to separate, the Kidney and Heart are said to have lost communication. This loss of communication is symbolized by Hexagram #12 of the I JING, "Disjunction". One common symptom associated with this loss of connection or capillary attraction is spermatorrhea in which the body loses its abiltiy to hold onto its JING or Yin Pure Essence. In other words, the capillary attraction between Fire and Water is broken and so the "Water" dribbles down as the Fire flares up. In women this often manifests as a particular types of leukorrhea.

Since the Yin is the Root of Yang, if the Yin becomes too weak, eventually the Yang will also collapse. In this case the Kidney Yin and Yang may both become Deficient. This often leads to the Kidney and Spleen Yang simultaneously becoming Deficient as in "Cock-crow" diarrhea. Since the Spleen is the Child of the Heart, if the Heart becomes weak, the Spleen may become Deficient for this reason as well. A dual Heart/Spleen Deficiency is not uncommon in clinical practice. In such cases, there are often symptoms of an unstable SHEN, poor digestion, Blood Deficiency, and the Spleen's inability to hold the Blood within its channels as in certain types of metrorrhagia. Since the Spleen is the main organ responsible for the generation of Blood, a simultaneous Spleen/Heart Deficiency can be a loop which is hard to break. Likewise, if the Spleen becomes weak, as the source of Postnatal Qi, it in turn will weaken the Kidneys, the source of Prenatal Qi. This then will only aggravate the relationship between the Kidneys, Liver, and Heart allowing the Heart Fire to burn further out of control.

Because the Heart and Lungs exist side by side in the Upper Burner, Deficiency or Heat in the one can aggravate Deficiency or Heat in the other. Deficiency of Upper Burner Qi is the same as Deficiency of ZONG or Chest Qi which in turn can lead to Chest BI or Obstruction, i.e. Stagnation of Qi and Blood in the Heart. Since Fire evaporates Yin, Deficient Fire in the Heart can contribute to the Lung Yin being weakened. Due to the special relationship between the Lungs and the Kidneys, if Lung Yin becomes Deficient, so most usually does Kidney Yin. If this happens, once again the Kidneys will be even less able to control the flaring of Heart Fire. Heat in the Upper Burner over time usually leads to Deficiency Cold in the Lower Burner. This can effect not only the Kidneys but the Bladder, Intestines, and the reproductive organs.

It is easy to see then that the flaring of Heart Fire and the weakening of the Kidneys can lead to a number of pathologic relations between the various organs, bowels, and humors of Chinese medicine. The practitioner and student of Chinese medicine will be able to further elucidate for themselves all the ramifications of this basic scenario. The number of named western diseases that can be caused by these various permutuations are numerous and include most of the "new" diseases such as AIDS, SLE, MS, etc. This basic scenario is what I believe the author of the 75th Difficulty of the NAN JING had in mind. The 75th Difficulty states: "If East (Liver) is Excess and West (Lung) is Deficient, disperse the South (Heart) and tonify the North (Kidneys)."[14] The OICS commentary on the NAN JING in interpreting this passage quotes the NEI JING: "One who does not understand this principle of treatment of the Emptiness is not justified in speaking of the treatment of complicated sicknesses."[15]

From the above discussion of the ramifications of Heart Fire on the other four solid organs, it is easy to see how Liu Wan-su in the Jin dynasty was led to believe that Fire is the supreme etiology of all disease. Although his overly simplistic theory of pathogenesis subsequently was proven to be incomplete, one of his ideas, the notion of Similar Transformation, is important in this discussion of flaring of Deficient Heart Fire. According to Liu Wan-su, since life is of the nature of Fire, any pathologic energy or substance in the body is likely to transform into Heat due to the influence of this basic Fire of Life. This is a case of the guest energy transforming into a similar energetic conformation as the basic host energy. As we shall see below, this theory of Similar Transformation will help us understand how this pathologic Fire is created in the first place.

The basic implication of our discussion so far is that Flaring of Heart Fire disturbs the SHEN or Mind and is the cause of the great majority of nervous and psychological disorders. In Traditional Chinese Medicine, the cause of mental disorders are divided into two general categories. They can either be Constitutional, i.e. Congenital, or Acquired. Constitutional etiologies include the transmission of Heat from the parents at conception, toxicity accumulated during gestation due to pollutants from either the environment or the mother's diet, the expectant mother's poor nutrition during pregnancy, or the mother's loss of emotional balance during pregnancy.

As discussed in THE PATH OF PREGNANCY, Chinese medicine believes that Heat can be transmitted at conception from either of the parents to the embryo. For this reason, the classics counsel that conception should not be allowed to take place within one hundred days of recuperating from a Hot disease. Chinese medicine also believes that toxins from the environment or from the mother's food can accumulate in the fetus. These are called TAI DU or "fetal toxins". Toxicity in Chinese medicine implies Heat. I have never heard of a Cold Toxin. Fetal Toxins usually result in and are discharged by such childhood disorders as measles and chickenpox. As discussed in TURTLE TAIL & OTHER TENDER MERCIES, if these Toxins are suppressed, they may develop into nervous (system) disorders, such as neurovascular headaches, eczema, and even Multiple Sclerosis. If the mother's diet is not adequate, the child may be born with congenitally insufficient Yin which will easily allow for insufficient Heart Blood, Flaring Fire in the Heart, and a disturbed SHEN. A case history of such a child has been presented by me in TURTLE TAIL. Chinese medicine also believes the child in utero is aware of the events transpiring around them, and, that due to the connection of the fetus to the mother's Heart through the CHONG MO, the child may easily be upset by emotional chaos and turmoil in the mother's life. One of the definitions of the child discussed in TURTLE TAIL is their inherently unstable SHEN. This instabiltiy extends back in utero. In other words, the child may be born with Flaring of Fire in the Heart due to their mother's emotional stress and strain.

Acquired or Postnatal mental disorders are due in general to an imbalance in Internal/External factors such as Exogenous pathogens, emotions, diet, sex, etc. including and especially severe and long-standing emotional strain. These injure the Qi and Blood or cause a loss of equilibrium between Yin and Yang. This results in the formation of any four of the following: 1) Phlegm, 2) Stagnant Qi, 3) Hyperactive Fire, and 4) Deficient Blood failing to nourish the Heart, i.e. the SHEN. Of these four etiologies, the first three are most commonly the culprits in the creation of mental disorder. Interestingly, due to Liu Wan-su's theory of Similar Tranformation, both Phlegm and Stagnant Qi have an innate tendency to transform into and aggravate pathologic Heat. This Heat then, over time, evaporates the Yin and/or the Blood.

In discussing Flaring of Liver Fire, Manfred Porkert describes the disease mechanism thus: "The energy flow of the oo. hepaticus et felleus (Liver & Gallbladder) is drastically reduced so that subsequent congestion leads to ardor ('glare'). This 'glare' is transported by the *qi* to the different body sites, possibly even to the top of the skull."[16] The symptoms of this include an "intensely colored tip and margins of the tongue; yellow or dry and sticky coating of the tongue; stringy and accelerated pulses (pp. chordales et celeri)."[17]

Previously I have said that a red-tipped tongue indicates Deficient Fire in the Heart. Here Manfred Porkert says that a red-tipped tongue can also be a symptom of Liver Fire. It is my opinion that most of the red-tipped tongues I see in my clinical practice begin, in fact, as Liver Qi Congestion. The Liver is called the "tempermental" organ in Chinese medicine.[18] It is the most easily affected organ by emotional sress and strain. Although classically it is said that the Liver is harmed by anger, any emotional stress will tend to "jam" the Liver.

Stress is intrinscially frustrating. We desire to do or accomplish or have more than we are able. This frustration is, in turn, a kind of anger. When we desire more than we can attain or manifest, the free flow and patency of our Qi is thwarted and becomes congested. Due to Similar Transformation, the accumulation of Stagnant Qi eventually becomes a Hot pathologic energy. Since Heat rises and since Fire has an affinity for the Heart, this Heat is easily transferred from the Liver to the Heart. Once this transfer takes place, a draft is created which fans the flames of the Liver and feeds the Fire in the Heart. This then most typically initiates the consumption of Kidney Yin.

Based on this scenario, the pulse that I find most typically associated with a red-tipped tongue amongst my patients makes perfect sense. What I find in the pulses of many such patients are a weak CUN position, this weakness being more pronounced on the left hand but also present on the right, a wirey quality, especially on the left GUAN, a thinner, threadier left pulse overall, and often a sunken quality on one or both CHIH positions. The weakness on the left CUN indicates Deficiency of the Heart. The thin left pulse overall suggests a systemic Yin Deficiency. The wirey left GUAN, often extending through the CHIH position, indicates Liver Congestion of Flaring. And the sunken CHIH positions indicate Kidney Deficiency. The pulse may be hurried or fast but since there is often a combination of Heat in the upper body with Cold in the lower, the pulse's speed may not accurately mirror the Heat. This depends on the relative predominance of Hot and Cold in such patients.

In understanding this conformation, it is useful to examine the pathological theories of two other of the Four Great Internists of the Jin-Yuan dynasties, Li Dong-yuan and Zhu Dan-xi, since both of these great masters, I believe, correctly explained significant factors contributing to this commonly encountered imbalance. Li Dong-yuan is the originator of the School of Postnatal Tonification, also known as the School of the Stomach/Spleen. Li Dong-yuan surmised that Internal Deficiency is the main cause of disease. Previous theoreticians had placed primary importance on Exogenous pathogens as the main cause of disease. But Li reasoned that if the Righteous Qi of the individual were strong, they would be relatively impervious to invasion. He emphasized that "poor diet, irregular living, and mental anguish depleted health"[19] since these exhaust the ZHENG or Righteous Qi. It was Li Dong-yuan who also first described the concept of Deficiency Fire. He arrived at this concept from Liu Wan-su's emphasis on Fire as the major cause of disease plus his own insight into the role of Deficient Righteous Qi.

Li Dong-yuan explained at length the concept of Yin Fire or YIN HUO. As Henry Lu explains: "Yin Fire refers to the fire generated by internal causes, including fatigue, consumption of foods, excessive joy or excessive anger or excessive worry or excessive contemplation, etc. and it belongs to the fire of the heart."[20] YIN HUO is further divided into two types: Excess and Deficient Fire. Excess Fire refers most usually to Fire due to an Exogenous pathogen. However, it can also be generated by Internal causes as well. Excess Fire most often attacks or is generated in the Stomach, Intestines, Liver, and Gallbladder. Deficient Fire is due to the exhaustion of True Yin. Li Dong-yuan also asserted that if the Stomach and Spleen become weak, Yin Fire may easily attack them and further disrupt their function.

These insights of Li Dong-yuan's are of great importance, especially at this time. We live in times not totally dissimilar from the Jin-Yuan dynasties which were a time of invasion, war, social and political upheaval, famine, stress, and great tension. Although in America our food is abundant in quantity, there is great doubt as to its vitality as witnessed by the popularity of vitamins and other dietary supplements. Due to processing, storage, pollution, adulteration, and preservatives, our diet does not, it seems, support our Righteous Qi adequately. This is compounded by our overconsumption of sweets, coffee, heavy red meats, spices, oils, and chilled foods and drinks, all of which further depress the Stomach/Spleen. Although weakness of the Stomach/Spleen is not, I believe, the main factor in the development of endemic Heat in the Heart, it is a contributing factor. It should also be noted that Li Dong-yuan not only habitually prescribed Stomach/Spleen tonifying herbs in his formulae but commonly included cooling herbs such as Coptis, Scutellaria, and Phellodendron to QING HUO, Clear Heat generated by Deficiency.

Zhu Dan-xi, having studied the theories of both Liu Wan-su and Li Dong-yuan, took their descriptions of the role of Fire as a pathogen and advanced them conceptually even further. As far back as the NEI JING, Chinese medicine had recognized two types of Righteous Fire functioning in the human organism. One is called Imperial or Monarch Fire. This is the True or Righteous Fire of the Heart. The other is called Ministerial or Auxilliary Fire. True Heart Fire is the Righteous Heat of the Heart. Ministerial Fire is primarily derived from the Lower Burner. Its root is the Kidney Fire, also called the Life Gate Fire or MING MEN HUO. Secondarily this Fire is associated with the Liver, Gallbladder, Triple Heater, Stomach, and Pericardium. It is the Ministerial Fire which is the foundation for all other Righteous Heat in the body. Especially it is the root of the Monarch Fire of the Heart. As Kiko Matsumoto puts it, "Ming Men is the small or supporting Fire that supports the Big Fire, the Heart..."[21] Although it is the vital Fire of Life, still it can also cause disease. It is because of this Fire that most pathogenic energies and substances transform into either pathologic Heat or Fire. This Fire both creates and should be transformed by the functioning of the organs, keeping in mind that the original connotation of the Chinese word HUA, transformation, was an alchemical one and not just a simple change.[22] As its best and most healthy expression, Ministerial Fire should transform into Light by the time it reaches the Heart, the Light of the Spirit, i.e. Enlightenment.

Zhu Dan-xi, in relating Fire to Yang, stated, "Yang energy is always in excess, whereas Yin energy is always in short supply."[23] This is a basic tenet of classical Chinese Yin/Yang theory. It is encountered in such diverse arts as FENG SHUI or Geomancy and abdominal palpation. In Geomancy, the East is Yang and the West is Yin. According to FENG SHUI, a location is appropriately balanced Yin to Yang if the Yang energy in the East, indicated by the features of the landscape, is proportional to the Yin energy of the West at a ratio of 3/5 to 2/5.[24] Likewise, in abdominal palpation, a palpable pulsing on the left side of the umbilicus is considered appropriate and a favorable prognostication. Whereas, a more prominent pulsation on the right side of the umbilicus, i.e. the Yin side of the body, is relatively unfavorable due to the "unnatural" occurence of the proportions of Yin to Yang this indicates.[25]

Zhu Dan-xi felt that the exhaustion of Yin was the main cause of Internally generated pathologic Fire. In other words, like Li Dong-yuan, he saw Deficiency Fire as being more of a problem than Excess Fire. However, unlike Li, Zhu felt that Deficiency of the Kidneys is more important than Deficiency of the Stomach/Spleen. Zhu Dan-xi's theory or school of thought is called the School of Watering Yin. Zhu said, "The Kidneys can hardly be filled up."[26] Therefore Zhu and his followers stressed the tonification of the Kidneys. "In his therapeutics, Chu (Zhu) advocated purging fire and nourishing yin."[27]

It is also important to note that although Zhu felt that Yin is by nature inherently Deficient as compared proportionally to Yang, certain behaviour would hasten its exhaustion and decline. Like his predecessor, Li Dong-yuan who thought that "Internal injury" was due to "intemperance in drinking and eating and overwork"[28], Zhu "thought indulgence was the root of all troubles."[29] What is usually overlooked in discussions of Zhu's work is that the second essential point in the theory of Watering Yin is that to maintain good health Zhu believed a person must remain physically active. "All creature are always active when they are in good health, and human beings are no exception. But the reason one can be active is that there is a sufficient amount of minister fire in the body."[30] In other words, Zhu did not seek to douse the body's Righteous Fire. He understood its importance as the very Fire of Life. What he saw, however, was that this Fire, due to intemperance and overindulgence, could burn out of control. "If kept in normal position, it would be helpful. If in reckless motion, it would injure the body."[31]

In the Ming dynasty, Xie Li-cai, Zhang Jing-yue, Zhao Zian-ke, and Li Zhong-zi combined the insights of Li Dong-yuan and Zhu Dan-xi in what has come to be known as the School of Warm Tonification. This is also known as the School of Prenatal Tonification. Although this school correctly saw the fundamental relationship between the Kidney Fire and the Middle Burner Fire and the importance of harmonizing Yin and Yang without undue attention being paid to the tonification of Yin, still, their routine use of warm herbs such as Cinnamon and Aconite to tonify the Kidney Yang may be dangerous in modern Americans who in general suffer from a hyperactive Ministerial Fire and a Deficiency of True Yin. Cortex Cinnamon is, for instance, traditionally contraindicated in Yin Deficiency with Internal Heat.[32] This is exactly what Zhou Ming-ying was referring to when she corrected my Cold BI formula. Since Heat, when it gets out of control, tends to burn up, it is true that over a long period of time or in extreme cases, the Lower Burner tends to become Cold while the Upper Burner becomes Hot. In such cases it is appropriate to use Zhang Jing-yue's warm tonification approach. However, this is not, in my experience, the commonly encountered situation at this time, though it may be in the future as the segment of the population between twenty and forty gets older.

In practical terms, the key point of this historical recapitulation of the development of the theory of pathologic Deficiency Heat in Chinese medical literature is the fact that this Heat is the result of immoderate behavior. It is my belief that the prevalence of the red-tipped tongue amongst young and middle-aged American adults and the Flaring of Heart Fire it signifies are due to our society's ever-accelerating overindulgence. In our search for a material solution to the main existential and spiritual problems of life, namely suffering and death, we have created a society and environment of run-away stress. Every new, technological solution has created further, even more complicated problems. These problems, whether they be personal, social, political, environmental, or moral can not be solved through technology and material "progress". The root problem is a spiritual one which can only be solved by a spiritual solution. In the meantime, all our efforts to extricate ourselves from our self-spun web of complexity only lead to further entanglement.

Each of us sees the problems of life from our own perspective. And each of us tends to emphasize our own perspective. For the nutritionist, our modern epidemic of chronic, degenerative diseases is due to denatured food and overconsumption of fats, sugars, simple carbohydrates, and stimulants. To the exercise physiologist, it is due to our lack of exercise and sedentary lifestyle. To the psychiatrist or psychotherapist, it is due to emotional stress and the artificiality of our interpersonal relationships. To the environmentalist, it is due to the presence of toxic pollutants and the exhaustion of pure natural resources such as fresh air, pure water, and adequate space. To the sociologist, it is due to overcrowding, lack of meaningful occupation, and the breakdown in our families and in the social compact. Each specialist has his or her own explanation for the accelerating degeneration of the quality of our lives and our health as a nation. However, such observations and criticisms are not currently fashionable. The majority of us have retreated into a Polyanna serendipity out of our total inability to deal with the stresses of modern life. Still, as a practitioner of Chinese medicine, I can confidently say that the red-tipped tongue is not going to go away simply because we hope it will.

The foremost implication for me of the red-tipped tongue is that we, as a society, are not able to cope with the stresses we have built into our lives. Most of us assume that we are reasonably healthy and that indeed we are coping as best we can. But the accumulation of Heat in the Heart belies that opinion. We assume that there is nothing we can do beyond what we are doing and if that is not enough, that's just too bad. In fact, many young and middle-aged adults who tried to turn their lives around and create a saner, healthier life for themselves and their society, have, due to exhaustion, given up and joined the ranks of the self-centered, immediate gratification, consumer society. In Boulder, known as a Mecca of alternative and holistic health, the opening of ice cream parlors, chocolate emporia, and French patisseries is more common than health-food stores. The only concession to health is a narcissistic preoccupation with maintaining a youthful exterior through frenetic activities like aerobics classes to the shouts of anorectic and amenorrheic coaches and Heart-pounding, Kidney-exhausting, rock music.

The stresses in our society are so pervasive as to go largely unnoticed. Our senses are constantly bombarded by stimulation. Many of us have become so over-heated that in fact we cannot tolerate silence or lack of stimulation. We are like motors stuck in high gear. Background music, movies, tv, magazines, newspapers, revealing and sexually provocative clothing, coffee, alcohol, drugs, traffic, the background hum of machinery, driving in cars, travelling in planes, artificial lighting, over-complex and over-flavored foods, unnatural situations without solutions, like the threat of nuclear annihilation, all assail us moment by moment. If one goes into retreat in a secluded, natural hermitage for even a month and then hears some rock 'n roll, one will understand the strength of its assault on our nervous systems which we never normally recognize. In China I have had young friends tell me that they dare not listen to rock 'n roll because it upsets them too much. It is our habituation to this stress that does not allow us to see it for how debilitating it is. Likewise, when the Ven. Dr. Trogawa Rinpoche came to America for the first time, he asked that his patients not drive to their diagnostic examination since the stress of driving would derange their pulses too much for accurate diagnosis. Rather than learning a great lesson from this request, his patients told him that in America such a request was a impossible demand even though 80% of them lived within two miles or a half hour's walk of the clinic.

Chinese medicine is not the only traditional medicine with a highly developed tongue diagnosis. Tibetan medicine, a cousin of Chinese medicine, likewise uses inspection of the tongue in making a diagnosis. Tibetan medicine has been thoroughly permeated by the Tibetan form of Buddhism, a highly developed system of analysing and manipulating the mind. Since Flaring of Heart Fire is due to mental imbalance and likewise causes mental imbalance, I believe practitioners of Traditional Chinese Medicine can gain a deeper understanding of the ramifications and treatment of this disorder by studying the Tibetan point of view on it. Tibetan medicine especially stresses life-style changes, diet, and "adjunctive" therapies which Chinese-style practitioners can add to their acupuncture and herbal treatment plans to make them even more effective. Also, the Tibetan description of this disorder is, perhaps, more engaging for the patient who may then participate in their treatment plan more "whole-heartedly".

According to both Ayurvedic and Tibetan medicine, redness of the front third of the tongue indicates derangement of the Wind or Air humor. This Wind (Tib. LOONG, Skt. VATTHA) is not exactly the same, yet also not totally dissimilar from the Chinese medical concept of Wind. Ayurvedic and Tibetan medicine posit three humors in the organism which must remain in dynamic balance if health is to be preserved. Wind or Air is one of these, the other two being Bile or Fire and Phlegm or Water. This concept of LOONG or Wind is further divided into five subdivisions. Wind is the energy which animates the body. Dr.

Trogawa says, "Wind is the working aspect of the Mind."[33] As such, it is almost identical to the Chinese concept of Qi. LOONG is the Tibetan translation of the Sanskrit PRANA which is likewise translated as Qi in Chinese. Although there are many different types of Wind disease according to Tibetan medicine, Wind imbalance is the primary etiology of all mental disorders. As Namkhai Norbu states in INTRODUCTION TO TIBETAN MEDICINE: "Mental illnesses are linked to alterations in this humor (Wind)."[34] Terry Clifford, author of TIBETAN BUDDHIST MEDICINE & PSYCHIATRY, reiterates this point when she says, "Of the three humours, wind is the one primarily associated with mental disturbances."[35]

Dr. Trogawa, in explaining the connection between Wind and the Mind, uses the analogy of a legless man riding a horse. The legless man is the Mind and the horse is the Wind. The Mind, in other words, is moved by the Wind. This Wind moves in the TSA. TSA means nerves, blood vessels, and energy pathways. They are analogous to the Chinese concept of JING MAI. Garma C.C. Chang explains, "Mind and prana (rLung, psychic energy) are two facets of one unity -- they should never be treated as two separate things. Mind is that which is aware; prana is the active energy which gives support to the awareness."[36] Clifford goes on to add that, "Although consciousness (and the life-force) is spread throughout the body, the 'owner' of it is the very subtle life-force in the life-vein at the heart."[37]

The relation between Wind, the Heart, and mental imbalance in Tibetan medicine is further clarified by Clifford: "The heart itself (sNying) is synonymous with mind in the Tibetan system; this is because consciousness, mental clarity, and the sense of self-identity arise from the heart center. Sensory input is carried by the all-pervasive Wind through the nerves or channels to the brain, where it is registered, but the consciousness relating to the sensory impressions and thoughts resides in the heart...It should be noted here that the results of disturbing the life-force at the heart are not only psychological but also physical. Wind in the heart produces stress disorders like high blood pressure and other cardiovascular diseases."[38]

The Wind or Air associated with the Heart is called SOK-LOONG or life wind. It is the first of the five types of Wind ennumerated in Tibetan medicine. Yeshe Donden describes the SOK-LOONG thus: "The life-sustaining wind is located in the crown of the head, and it mainly circulates or functions from that area through-out the chest. With respect to its functions, it enables swallowing of food, respiration (inhaling and exhaling of air), spitting out saliva, and sneezing. It provides clarity to one's mind and to the sensory organs and holds life in the sense that it provides the physical basis for life to lodge itself."[39] Derangement or imbalance of the Life-wind is so completely identified with mental imbalance in Tibetan medicine and culture that madness is simply called SOK-LOONG. As Garma C.C. Chang says, "In fact, intense neurotic behavior and the psychological and physiological symptoms of nervousness are called simply the 'sok-lung', a disorder of life-wind."[40]

There are two basic stages in the development of a Wind disorder. The first is augmentation. That is, the humour Wind becomes Excessive vis a vis the other two humours. Epstein and Rabgay list the factors responsible for the aggravation and augmentation of Wind disease as follows:

1) poor diet (e.g. excessive bitter, light, or coarse foods, such as coffee, cucumber, strong tea, or pork)

2) excessive sexual intercourse

3) insufficient food or prolonged fasting

4) insomnia

5) phsyical, oral, or mental strain or exertion on an empty stomach

6) obsessive thoughts ("thinking about something for a long time without actually doing something about it")

7) hemorrhage

8) excessive vomiting or diarrhea

9) exposure to cold such as breezes

10) lack of appetite

11) excessive joy or sadness

12) depression (especially as a result of frustrated desires)

13) malnutrition (insufficient protien)

14) straining in passing excreta, forceful retention of excreta, excessive forceful sneezing or spitting[41]

In reviewing this list, the Chinese-trained practitioner will recognize a number of factors which similarly could be explained as causing a Flaring Heart Fire and Deficiency of Kidney Yin. Coffee and tea weaken Kidney Yin, stimulate the MING MEN HUO, stimulate the SHEN, and irritate the Liver. Zhu Dan-xi said that excess sex is a main cause of Kidney Yin Deficiency. Fasting consumes Yin substance in general. Insomnia, often caused by Yin Deficiency, likewise leads to Yin Deficiency and an agitated SHEN. Any exertion when Stomach Qi is at a low ebb may adversely deplete reserve energy stored in the Kidneys, i.e. the JING, a species of Yin Qi. Obsessive thinking disturbs the Liver/HUN and therefore the SHEN and weakens the Middle Burner, the Postnatal root of Qi and Blood. Hemorrhage, diarrhea, and vomiting all cause Fluid Deficiency which leads to Blood and/or Yin Deficiency. Exposure to cold harms the Kidneys by depleting the MING MEN HUO; whereas exposure to Wind elevates Liver Yang. Lack of appetite in the sense of anorexia nervosa is, in Chinese medicine, most often due to Liver Qi Congestion leading to Heart Fire and Deficient Kidney Yin.[42] Excessive joy or anger qualify as unrestraint of the Seven Passions in Chinese terminology and adversely affect primarily the Heart, Liver, and Kidneys.[43] Insufficient protein means lack of Yin-tonifying foods, such as eggs, fish, dairy, and organ meats. The last etiology on this list, straining at passing stools, etc., means that one is either thwarting the regular flow of Qi or unnaturally pressuring its flow, both of which may result in Qi Stagnation, eventually of the Liver and eventually transforming into Heat.

The second stage in a Wind disorder is when the unnaturally augmented Wind flows into an inappropriate channel, thus displacing one of the other Winds. Wind by nature has a tendency to rise. Each of the five Winds is stacked on the Wind below it. If one Wind becomes augmented, it will flow up perversely into another Wind's territory. One way of diagnosing a Wind derangement in

Tibetan medicine is the detection of an unnaturally strong palpitation of the abdominal aorta above the navel. The higher up this palpitation can be felt the more serious the displacement or derangement of the Winds. A healthy LOONG should cause pulsing of the abdominal aorta to be felt primarily at the umbilicus. In Chinese medicine, upper abdominal palpitation of the descending aorta usually indicates a Righteous Qi Deficiency in general and in particular a Yin Deficiency of the Kidneys.[44] The Wind that is most susceptible to displacement by perversion of upwardly rebelling Wind, to use familiar Chinese terminology, is the SOK-LOONG or Life-wind.

Symptoms associated in Tibetan medicine with a pathologic augmentation of Wind are susceptibilty to cold and shivering, especially under stress, a tendency to lose weight, diffuse pain on movement in all part of the body, frequent but incomplete defecation, pale or bluish urine, restlessness, sighing, tinnitus, vertigo, insomnia, erratic and diffuse pains, increased talking, loss of strength, loss of clarity of one or more of the senses, borborygmus, abdominal distention, anger, yawning, a frequent desire to stretch, muscle cramping, fornication, backache, chest pain, irritability, a dry, red, rough tongue, and a weakish, superficial pulse. A patient with not only Excess Wind but also derangement in its flow will exhibit even more restlessness. When sitting down, he will want to stand up. When standing up, he will want to move. He will begin to whistle, drum his fingers, or fidget. As the mind begins to flutter, the symptoms of tinnitus, chest and upper back pain, palpitations of the Heart, and chest distress and oppression will increase. The patient will make chronic verbal slips, decision making becomes difficult, and when writing he will make many errors.

This list of symptoms is a compilation based on the oral teachings of Dr. Trogawa and a list which appears in "Mind and Mental Disorders in Tibetan Medicine" by Epstein and Rabgay.[45] As in our discussion of the etiology of Wind disorders, I believe the experienced Chinese medical clinician will be able to account for the majority of these symptoms using the classical theories of pathogenesis described above. If Wind disorders are allowed to progress unchecked or untreated, their aggravation may result in madness or insanity. In English language texts on Chinese medicine, this constellation of symptoms is diagnosed as neurasthenia, a diagnosis, according to Ted Kaptchuk, which has been formally abolished by western MDs but which is a category I believe to be quite useful in contemporary clinical practice.[46] In Chinese, neurasthenia is usually referred to as SHEN JING. ACUPUNCTURE: A COMPREHENSIVE TEXT, in discussing neurasthenia, says: "In Chinese medicine, the symptoms associated with this condition include depression, palpitations, insomnia, lassitude, spermatorrhea, and others. It is attributed to weakness and disruption of the Heart, Liver, Spleen, or Kidney Qi. The Depletion of the Kidney Yin may cause Fire in the Heart to flare upward and the Liver Yang to become Excessive ... Treatment is directed towards calming the Heart's Spirit, strenghtening the Kidneys, and regulating the Liver and the Spleen."[47]

According to Tibetan medical theory, the three humors, Wind, Bile, and Phlegm, are not naturally equal in proportion. The normal proportions of these fluctuate in a cyclic way acording to the seasons of the year, age of the patient, environment, and astrologocal influences. "For example, young people up to the age of sixteen are prone to disorders of the Phlegm, whereas the adult is more inclined to disturbances of Bile and the old to illness linked to Air."[48] This is because there is proportionally more of each of these humors during these stages of life. If in adults one would expect a predominance of Bile disease, why is there an epidemic pathologic predominance of Wind in Americans up to forty years of age? As noted above, Wind imbalance in Tibetan medicine closely corresponds to Flaring of Heart Fire with attendant Yin Deficiency. One of Zhu Dan-xi's important observations is that aging is linked to the depletion of Kidney Yin which thus gives rise to Deficient Heat.

The implication is that young Americans are burning ourselves out prematurely. We have been bombarded with so much sensory input and stimulation that we are prematurely exhausting our True Yin. On the other hand, we as a generation may have been Congenitally Deficient and our SHEN may have been agitated at birth due to the trauma and turmoil of World War II. Certainly surveying the ears of young Americans from twenty to forty suggests that this generation is Congenitally Deficient, if in fact the shape of the ear is an indication of Prenatal vigor or XIAN TIAN QI as some schools of Oriental medicine believe. It seems to me that far too many Americans this age have small or no earlobes with very thin outer helixes and that their ears are placed relatively high on the head. On the other hand, a junk food diet as children, tv, radio, movies, rock 'n roll, the turmoil of the sixties and seventies, drugs, cars, the breakdown of the family, early and excessive sex, etc., etc. all seem to have taken their toll.

On top of this, or as an explanation of this, Tibetan Buddhist medicine also posits the existence of large cycles of time or eons which also have an effect on the preponderance of the humors of those beings living in those cycles. These are astrological or biorhythmic influences on a truly vast scale. According to Tibetan Buddhism, we are living in the KALI YUGA or NYIK-MAI DU, the Iron or Degenerate Age. Tibetan Buddhism posits that we and our world are in a cosmic decline, that the ZEITGEIST is one of degeneracy and decay on all levels. Traditonally the astrological scriptures, such as the KALACHAKRA TANTRA or WHEEL OF TIME, describe five decays inherent in this age which include the physical universe, the beings within that world, and even time itself. Not only are the contents and the container, i.e. the beings and the world they inhabit, degenerating on the physical level, but we are also degenerating on an emotional and moral level as well. This is the Buddhist explanation for our escalating and myriad modern problems, from pollution to the appearance of new and recalcitrant diseases such as AIDS, Toxic Shock Syndrome, Lou Gehrig's Disease, and many forms of cancer. This deterioration of the KALI YUGA is described as a speeding up of everything eventually leading to "spontaneous combustion" and apocalypse. According to Namkhai Norbu, a Tibetan Lama Doctor living and teaching in Italy, we have about three hundred years before the KALI YUGA "bottoms out".[49] It appears to me that our contemporary generation is likewise "stuck in high gear" and over-heating.

According to Buddhism, nothing can be done to prevent this inexorable progression on a cosmic level. Just as we can not stop the arrival of fall and winter, nor in fact should we even attempt to, the KALI YUGA and its over-heating and exhaustion are a natural manifestation of this part of the universe's old age. Our premature burnout or Wind imbalance mirrors the tone of the times.

This does not mean, however, that as individuals we can not minimize and treat the ill effects of this ZEITGEIST in ourselves and in our patients. Guru Padmasambhava, at the same time as prophesying the various decadences of the KALI YUGA, also suggested ways the impact of these could be mitigated. As human beings, we have the intelligence to recognize the pattern within which we find ourselves. Because of this intelligence, we can work with our situation in a skillful way, using this term in its Buddhist sense.[50] To use the Chinese concept, as humans we cannot resist the will of Heaven and Earth, but as humans we can, by defining that will, use it to our own advantage within certain limits. Like a sailboat tacking against the wind, we cannot fly in the face of the cycle of change in which we live, but neither are we helpless with nought to do but run before it.

The Chinese therapeutic principles for treating Flaring of Heart Fire with Deficiency of Kidney Yin are to Regulate the Qi, Calm the SHEN, Clear the Heart, and Tonify the Deficiency. The systems most commonly addressed are the Heart, which stores and supports the SHEN, the Liver, which distributes the regular and rhythmic flow of Qi, and the Kidneys, the root of the Heart and the repository of the Marrow which in Chinese medicine encompasses the Central Nervous System including the brain, the SUI HAI or Sea of Marrow. These systems may be treated with either herbs or acupuncture, or, from my point of view, preferably with a combination of both.

If acupuncture is to be used, the more distal a point is on the extremity the more effective it tends to be for treating the mental aspects of its associated organ's imbalance. Also certain points have a well-defined and verified effect on the SHEN and such points become increasingly more important in this age of mental stress. A Colorado acupuncturist who apprenticed with an exceedingly perceptive and profound Chinese doctor was told by his teacher that almost all Americans should be needled at SHEN MEN (Ht 7) during the course of their treatment for almost any ailment. SHEN MEN, as the Earth point on the Fire meridian, is the Sedation point of the Heart. It naturally disperses any pathologic accumulation of Heat in that organ. It is also the YUAN Source point of the Heart and therefore it simulataneously balances the Yin and Yang of the Heart by accessing the YUAN QI which, interestingly, is primarily associated with the Kidneys.

NEI GUAN (Per 6) is also a very important point for the treatment of all Heart and chest disorders, especially if there is physical symptomology, such as palpitations or pain, as well as mental. The Hand JUE YIN regulates the Liver function in the Upper Burner, effects the Heart directly, and is also associated with the regulation of MING MEN HUO and the transformation of Kidney Fire into the Light of the Spirit. The meanings implied in the name XIN BAO, Heart Wrapper, and in the term JUE YIN, both as an identity and as a description, and the European insight in naming this meridian Circulation/Sex all deserve thought in understanding the functions of points on this channel.

Besides SHEN MEN and NEI GUAN, I also believe that American acupuncturists should pay more attention to the differential use of the other distal points on the Hand SHAO YIN and JUE YIN meridians and should not just use SHEN MEN and NEI GUAN in every case of emotional upsetment. For instance, LAO GONG (Per 8) is not only indicated for more extreme mental agitation than NEI GUAN but also is particularly indicated if there is a sensation of Qi rising to the top of the body.[51] Points on the head, such as BAI HUI (GV 20) and YIN TANG, are also powerful for calming the Spirit and sedating overactive Yang. However, these points should be used more for extreme cases where mental derangement is severe. This is especially so for BAI HUI.

Dr. Trogawa says that according to the MEN-NGAK or secret oral tradition on the teaching of TSA-LOONG THIG-LE, Tibetan pranayama yoga, BAI HUI should not be needled with impunity. This point is the terminal point of the central spiritual axis and inexpert manipulation of this point may have subtle and long-lasting negative effects on the SOK-LOONG. Rather the Tibetan esoteric yogic tradition advises needling what the Chinese call SI SHEN CONG. These are four points located one CUN on each of the four sides of BAI HUI. However, as we will discuss below, indirect moxabustion at BAI HUI may be very helpful in treating mental problems as long as they are not associated with high blood pressure.

My experience and the advise of Ted Kaptchuk[52] is that mental problems, unless they are severe, should not be needled more than once per week. Since they are at such a deep level, we can say that the patient does not have Flaring of Heart Fire but is Flaring of Heart Fire. Therefore, successful treatment means changing how a person experiences themself and reality at a deep level. If this change is imposed upon one too fast, the patient wil recoil from the treatment. In Tibetan medicine great importance is placed on treating a patient slowly over a long period of time. In our hurry-up world where the doctor is just as likely to suffer from a red-tipped tongue as the patient, patience is sometimes difficult, but it is of utmost importance if real and lasting results are to be achieved. Similarly, it is also my opinion that not too many points should be used during any one treatment in the treatment of mental/emotional disorders. The energy of the patient is already scattered and it should not be pulled in too many directions at one time. In such situations, less is often more, and the acupuncturist is advised to think deeply about the nature of each point chosen. Wherever one point can do the work of two or more, this is the point that should be used.

Using Chinese-style acupuncture, points should also be selected on the Foot TAI YANG and the DU MO channels. Both of these channels enter the brain and have a definite effect on the Central Nervous System. Also it is wise not to forget the outer line of Foot TAI YANG points on the back. Many of the points on this outer line are SHU or Associated points regulating the spiritual aspect of the associated organ. According to Kok Yuen-leung, the SHEN which resides in the Heart has its reflection in each of the other four solid organs. PO HU (Bl 42) is the Associated point of the PO. This is the aspect of the SHEN residing in the Lungs which directs the physical energies of the YING, WEI, and Blood. SHEN TANG (Bl 44) is the Associated point of the SHEN itself. HUN MEN (Bl 47) is the Associated point of the HUN. The HUN is the aspect of the SHEN which directs the thought process and resides in the Liver. YI SHE (Bl 49) is the Associated point of the YI. This is the aspect of the SHEN which directs the process of recollection and reflection. It resides in the Spleen. And finally, ZHI SHI (Bl 52) is the Associated point of the Will which resides in the Kidneys. These points, with the exception of ZHI SHI, are seldom met with in clinical practice since contemporary Traditional Chinese Medicine tends to downplay the spiritual and esoteric aspect of its

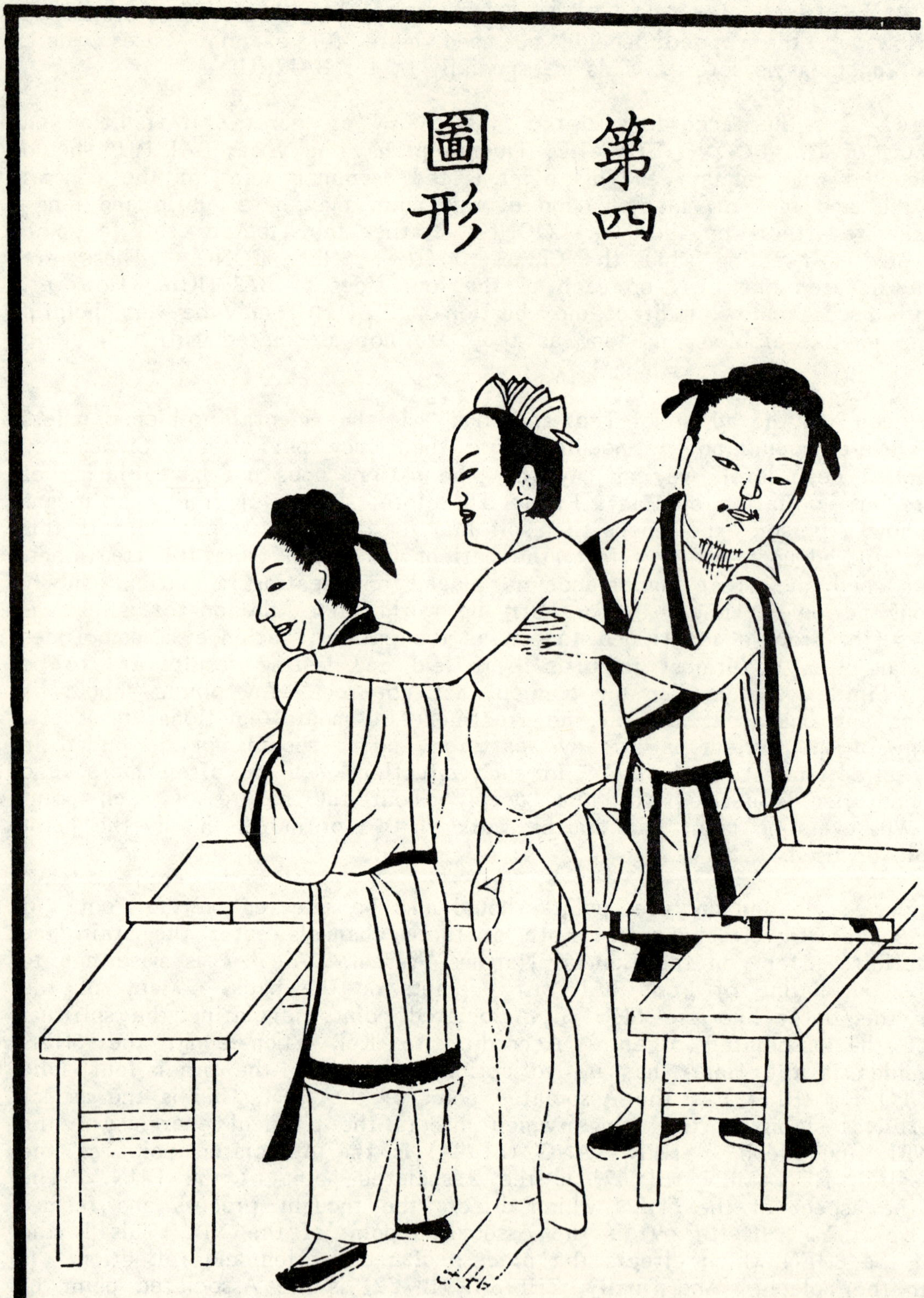
第四圖形

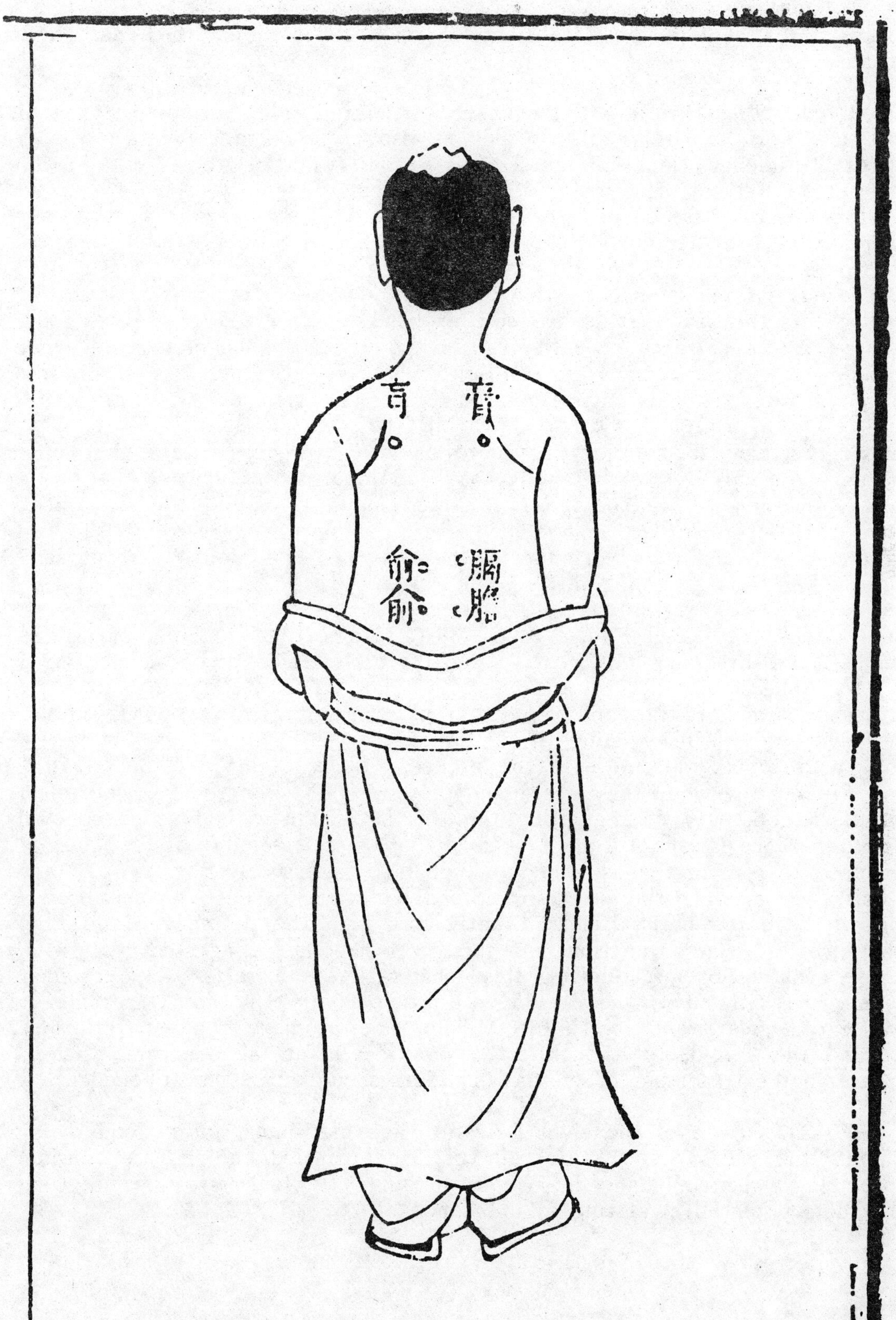
膏肓
膈俞
膽俞

heritage. However, in the treatment of mental disorders, they deserve more attnetion.

GAO HUANG SHU (Bl 43) is the back Associated point of the "Space Below the Heart", i.e. the vital center. This is also an important point in the treatment of Deficiency Heat in the Upper Burner whether this Heat be in the Lungs or the Heart. This point is also contemporaneously often overlooked in clinical practice. The concept of the GAO HUANG is hazy at best in modern Traditional Chinese Medicine. It is my belief that it refers to the place in the chest where the SOK-TSA or Life-vein which supports the SOK-LOONG is located and thus its importance in the classics. The ancients believed that if an Evil Qi enters this space it is difficult at best to cure and severely affects the life-force of the patient.[53] Although this point can be needled, traditionally it was more often moxaed even for Deficiency Heat. Chuang Cho, during the Jin dynasty, wrote a famous monograph on the application of moxa on this point called GAO HUANG JIU FA or THE METHOD OF MOXABUSTION AT GAO HUANG. Lu and Needham, citing more modern literature, state that moxa at this point is useful in treating pulmonary tuberculosis, bronchitis, pleurisy, neurasthenia, and general weakness, all of which may be caused by Yin Deficiency Heat in the Upper Burner.[54] Included are two ilustrations showing the location of GAO HUANG and its treatment by moxabustion, one from the Southern Song and the other from the Ming dynasty.

Points on the Hand and Foot YANG MING are effective for treating mental problems since dispersing the YANG MING is an efficient way of clearing Heat. The YANG MING are by nature Excess.[55] The YANG MING have an important relationship with both Pre and Postnatal Qi. The Large Intestine is involved in the production of Kidney Yang through the Internal Duct of the Triple Heater. The Stomach, of course, initiates the process of the creation of YING QI. The bowels are healthy when they are unobstructed.[56] Keeping the bowels open and moving is a good way of regulating the Qi of the entire body and especially of holding rebellious Qi down. In traditional Japanese medicine, it is believed that a tendency to constipation is linked to high blood pressure, apoplexy, and arteriosclerosis.[57] Certainly there is a reciprocal relationship between the bowels and the Liver since the peristalsis is directly linked to the patiency of Qi flow due to the Liver's dredging function. If the Liver becomes congested, this will tend to cause constipation and relieving this constipation is a reflex way of smoothing Liver Qi. HE GU (LI 4) and ZU SAN LI (St 36) Calm the mind, Disperse pathologic Heat, Regulate and Tonify the Middle, and promote the separation of the Clear and the Turbid. Although these points are an acupuncture cliché, still their use in the treatment of mental disorders should not be overlooked.

The CHONG MO, one of the eight Extraordinary meridians, in my opinion closely resembles the SOK-TSA or Life-vein of Tibetan medicine if we consider its symptomology when imbalanced. Woolerton and McClean give the following list of disorders potentially relating to imbalance of the CHONG MO:

Digestive ulcers
Gastric ulcers
Hyperacidity
Gynecological disorders
Low back pain

Palpitations
Stomachache
Heart disease in general[58]

In classical Chinese medicine, the eight Extraordinary meridians are usually used in pairs, the CHONG MO being paired with the YIN WEI MO. Each of the eight Extraordinary meridians has a master or command point. Most often the command points of the paired Extraordinary meridians are used in tandem. NEI GUAN, which we have discussed above, is the command point of the YIN WEI MO. The command point of the CHONG MO is GONG SUN (Sp 4). I believe that these points are very useful in treating disorders associated with a red-tipped tongue.

In the ZHEN JIU DA CHENG there is a discussion of the use of the eight Extraordinary meridians. Yang Ji-zhou recommends in treating CHONG MO related problems the practitioner should first needle GONG SUN. The general indications given for this point vis a vis its "command" function are: the "nine types" of Heart disorders, knotted chest, stagnant and upset Stomach, accumulation of food and drink in the Stomach, intestinal rumbling, diaphragmatic disturbances, umbilical pain, abdominal soreness, distention of the sides, various types of "malaria", acute Heart pain, retained palcenta, confusion, and diarrhea. Yang goes on to list a score or so of combinations of other points to needle after needling GONG SUN and NEI GUAN to treat a variety of complaints and problems.[59] I believe these combinations should be considered when treating patients with a red-tipped tongue.

The CHONG MO is the deepest, most fundamental channel in the body. It is sometimes called the JING HAI or Sea of the Twelve Meridians. When using the command points of the eight Extraordinary meridians, which Kiko Matsumoto believes develop embryologically before the so-called organ meridians, it is my opinion that one should take into account their astrological availability according to the LING GWEI PA FA, the Spiritual Turtle Eight Methods. This will, in my experience, maximize the benefits of the treatment. According to this system of point selection, if one command point of a paired couple is "open", the other paired point is also accessible. In other words, if according to the Spiritual Turtle calculations NEI GUAN is open at a particular hour of a particular day, then GONG SUN is also open. This dual availability makes this system more clinically flexible.

The Chinese herbal treatment of Flaring of Heart Fire with Deficient Kidney Yin is more complex than its acupuncture treatment. There are a number of herbs which calm the Spirit. Some of these, such as Radix Salvia miltorrhiza, Semen Zizyphus spinosae, Spirit of Poria, Arillus longana, Semen Biotae, Radix Polygalae, and Caulis Polygoni multiflori, calm the Heart by tonifying the Heart Blood or Heart Yin. Others, such as Cinnabar, Dragon Bone, Pearl, Oyster Shell, and Magnetite, weigh down the fluttering Spirit. The first group calm the Spirit by nurturing the Heart; whereas the second group directly sedate the Spirit by restraining it. Radix Ophiopogonis, Radix Angelica sinensis, Bulbus lilli, and both cooked and raw Radix Rehmanniae also tonify the Blood and Yin, although Chinese medicine does not ascribe to these the specific function of calming the SHEN. They are often included in formulae for Flaring of Heart Fire to nurture the Yin of the Kidneys, Liver, and Heart.

Herbs for clearing pathologic Fire in the Heart include Rhizoma Coptidis, Embryo of Lotus Seed, Fructus Forsythia, raw Radix Glycyrrhizae, Herba Lopthatheri, Caulis Akebiae, Medulla Junci, etc. However one must be careful in using these herbs. If the Kidney Yang or the Middle Burner Fire are weak due to prolonged or pronounced dysfunction of the other organs, these herbs are contraindicated. Interestingly, the last three mentioned above, Clear Heat in the Heart by dispersing the Small Intestine through diuresis. Instead, Radix Phellodendron, Radix Anemarrhenae, and other herbs which lower Deficient Fire by primarily tonifying the Yin should be used.

As for formulae, there are many that can be modified to fit the various symptoms and conformations which may arise along with pathologic Heat in the Heart as indicated by a red-tipped tongue. Free and Easy Decoction (XIAO YAO TANG) can be modified to treat a large number of gynecological/emotional disorders, such as insomnia, constipation, menopausal hot flashes, migraines, skin lesions, PMS, dysmenorrhea, and vaginitis. Restoring the Spleen Decoction (GUI PI TANG) can be modified to treat combined Spleen/Heart Deficiency disorders such as insomnia, menorrhagia, metrorrhagia, palpitations, anxiety, chronic vascular headaches, allergies, thrombocytopenic purpura, leukemia, chronic Pelvic Inflammatory Disease, etc. And Heavenly Emperor Heart Tonic Elixir (TIAN WANG BU XIN TAN) can be modified to treat insomnia, palpitations, neurosis, and anxiety. If it is taken with CHIH PAI PA WEI WAN, it treats Heart Deficiency with relatively more Heat and Kidney weakness. Symptoms may include spermatorrhea, palpitations, skin lesions, polyuria, nocturia, chronic cystitis, herpes genitalia, etc. If TIAN WANG BU XIN TAN is taken with Lycium Rehmannia Pills (JI JU DI HUANG WAN), it is indicated for Heart palpitations, dream-disturbed sleep, nervousness, headaches, urinary weakness, decline of vision, night blindness, and hypertension.

A complete explication of the herbal formulae for treating all the various manifestations of Deficient Heat in the Heart is beyond the scope of this work. However, the main point of this piece is that, although a red-tipped tongue has become almost standard in young American adults, it should not be discounted. Herbal formulae for such patients should take the implications of the red-tipped tongue into account both in terms of the choice of the basic formulae and in the selection of the individual ingredients. Since herbs are, in my opinion, better suited for tonifying Yin than acupuncture, they should be a prominent part of any treatment plan for disorders associated with this diagnostic sign.

In my practice I use a combination of herbal formulae and acupuncture. However I do not just simply duplicate my herbal treatment with an energetically identical acupuncture treatment. I believe that it is easier to tonify with herbs than with acupuncture and, as stated above, particularly the Blood and Yin. Acupuncture is more effective for dispersing Excess and also for balancing the flow of Qi. Therefore my approach is to prescribe herbal formulae to tonify the Blood and Yin and to use acupuncture to help in the speedy relief of symptoms which are caused by Excess, both local and systemic. Once these symptoms have been remedied, I continue herbal treatment alone for some time, usually switching from custom-blended, bulk herbs to patent medicines as the condition becomes more stabilized. Then, once the Yin energies are relatively more replete, I once again use acupuncture to keep the patient in balance. At this stage, I generally do not use ZANG FU syndrome correlated needle formulae but utilize acupuncture protocols based entirely on the flow of Qi and its transformation as revealed by Wang Shu-he's system of pulse diagnosis. This is an acupuncturist's acupuncture, not the "herbalized" acupuncture of modern TCM.

The treatment of the various disorders which arise as variations of this scenario of Flaring MING MEN HUO affecting the Heart and Liver usually require more than just herbs and acupuncture to effect a cure which will last over time. Although Chinese adjunctive therapies, such as diet, exercise, and meditation are good beginnings in fleshing out a complete treatment plan, Tibetan medicine, due to its more complete and extensive description of this problem and its emphasis on life-style, offers an even more comprehensive treatment.

One of the indications in Tibetan medicine for the use of moxabustion is the treatment of mental/emotional problems due to Wind. In Chinese medicine, many practitioners might tend to shy away from using moxa with a red-tipped tongue just as Zhou Ming-ying was afraid of using Aconite with my knee patient. In general, moxa is contraindicated in Hot diseases. However, this is a Deficiency Heat and moxa can be safely and effectively used in its treatment as long as the tongue is not also coated with a substantial yellow fur. Unless the patient is psychotic, indirect moxa is usually sufficient. We have discussed the classical Chinese use of moxa at GAO HUANG SHU to treat Deficiency Heat in the upper Burner above. Tibetan medicine not only suggests the use of moxa in treating psychological problems but has identified a number of specific points which help restore balance to the Winds and especially to the SOK-LOONG. These can be moxaed by the patient or their family at home in between office visits or instead of office visits if the course of treatment is to stretch over a prolonged period of time, which is often the case in such cases. The following is a brief synopsis of some of these Tibetan moxa points for the treatment of psychoemotional disorders.

LOONG-SANG means Wind point. It is located on the tip of the spinous process of the seventh cervical vertebra. It is flanked bilaterally by two adjunctive points of the same name and indications. These are located one Tibetan CUN, i.e. one thumb width, to either side of the central point. These adjunctive points are used in conjunction with the central point in the treatment of more severe cases. The adjunctive or flanking points are more nearly identical to the Chinese HUA TO JIA JI points than to the Bladder SHU points which are 1/2 CUN further lateral. The Tibetan indications for moxa at this point are extreme nervousness, neurosis, hysteria, palpitations, insomnia, and headache due to Wind imbalance. In such cases this point will usually be sore to palpation.

The back SOK-TSA points (SOK-TSA GYAB-SANG) are located on the tip and one Tibetan CUN to the right and left of the spinous process of the fifth thoracic vertebra. These points can be moxaed if the Wind has erroneously entered the Life-vein or SOK-TSA. They treat agitation, trembling, neurosis, psychosis, and "water retention around the Heart due to worry, suffering, etc."[60]

The Great Point of the Heart (NYING-SANG CHEN-MO) is located on the ventral centerline three Tibetan CUN below the Chinese point TIAN TU (CV 22) in the suprasternal notch. Moxa at this point treats palpitations, great sorrow, a feeling of emptiness, and emotional upsetment resulting in an inability to eat or to digest one's food properly.

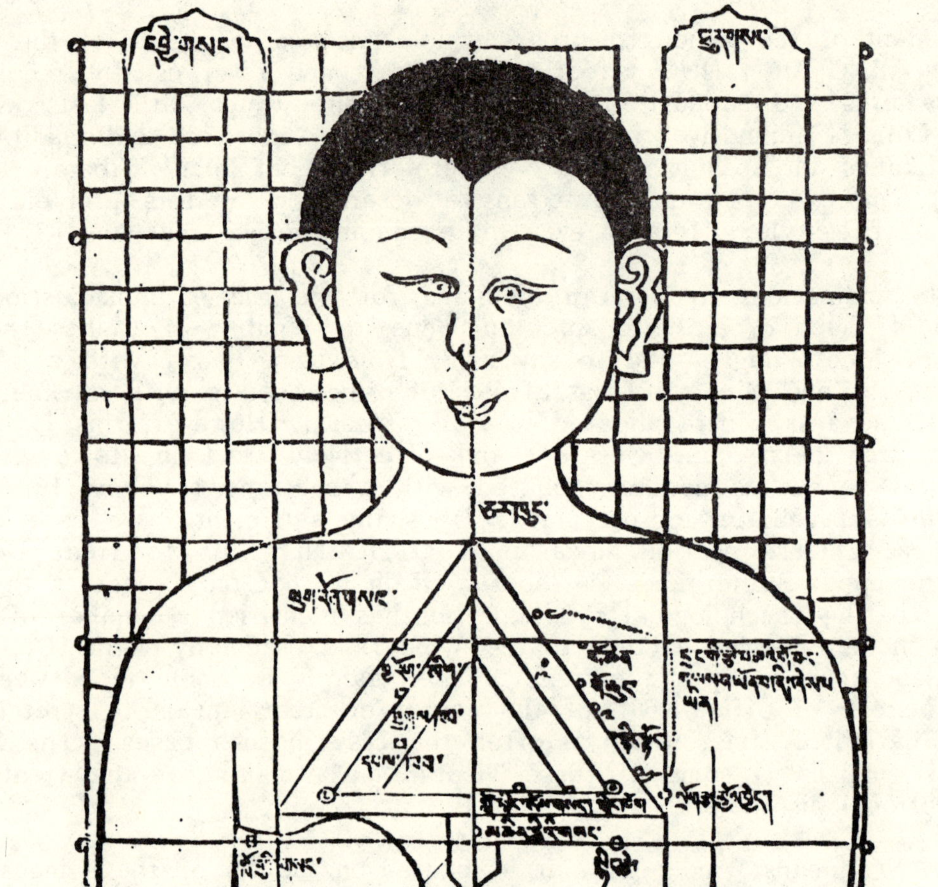

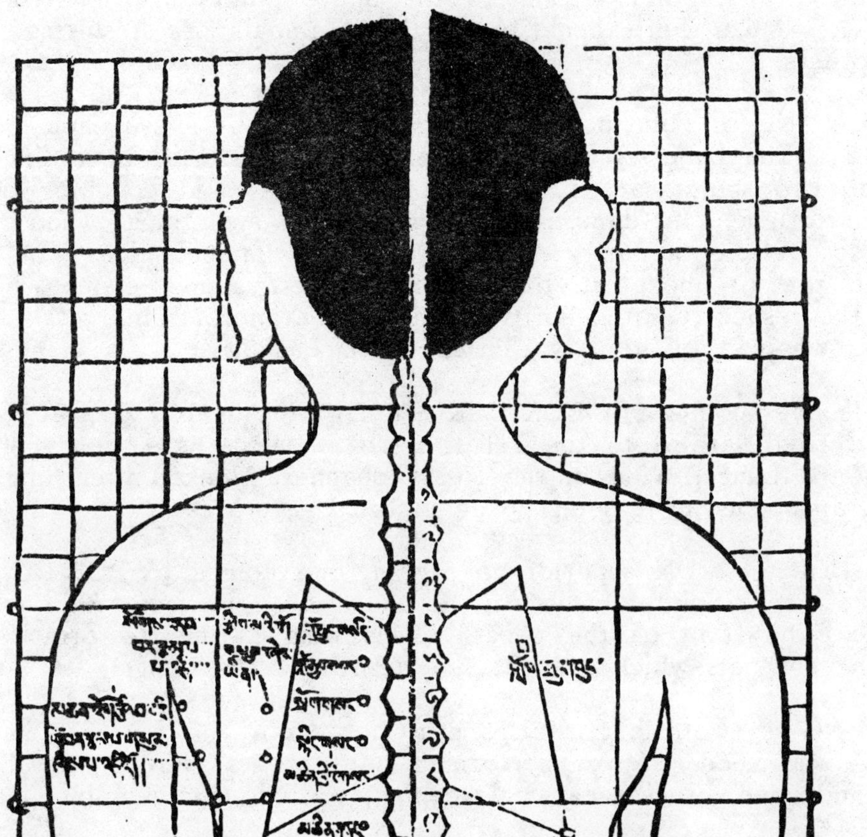

The Life-wind point (SOK-LOONG SANG) is located bilaterally two Tibetan CUN to the Chinese point SHAN ZHONG (CV 17) and one CUN superior. Moxa here treats nervous disorders due to Wind resulting in agitation.

One Tibetan CUN further lateral to the above points are located the LO-WAI BAR-SANG. Moxa here benefits all Wind imbalances resulting in Lung and Heart disorders.

The THUK-SANG or Mind points are located one CUN above each of the LO-WAI BAR-SANG. The benefits of moxa at these points are, according to Namkhai Norbu, relief of pulmonary inflammation, dyspnea, and coughing due either to exertion or fatigue. In Chinese terminology these symptoms, when taken together, are due to Deficient Yin. Although Norbu Rinpoche does not mention any psychiatric use of moxa at these points, their name cannot be accidental. THUK is the respectful or honorific term in Tibetan for mind. A Realized person has THUK; whereas an ordinary sentient being has SEM.

The Crow's Eyes points (JA-ROK MIK-SANG) are located one CUN superior and one CUN further lateral to the THUK-SANG. Moxa here treats disturbances of the Heart and Lungs, Wind in the Heart channel, blocked breathing, short, rapid breathing, and pains as if being poked in the Heart area.

Going one Tibetan CUN superior yet again, one comes to BUP-RON SANG, the Complete & Fresh points. One can do moxa here to treat pain travelling from the back to the front of the chest. This pain is due to erratic Wind having entered the channels which connect the Heart and the Lungs.

TSHAG-SANG is two Tibetan CUN posterior from the anterior hairline on the midline of the head. Moxa performed here treats pain in the brain, vertigo, epilepsy, and Wind diseases causing weeping, wailing, and jumping up and down.

The locations and indications for these points as used in Tibetan medicine are based on ME-TSAI LAK-LEN SHAY-GYI ME-LONG (THE CRYSTAL MIRROR OF THE PRACTICE OF MOXABUSTION) by Namkhai Norbu and on Namkhai Norbu's oral commentary to this text.[61] The accompanying Tibetan blockprint illustrations show the locations of some of these points. According to Terry Clifford, the spinous processes corresponding to LOONG-SANG and SOK-TSAI GYAP-SANG will become sore to the touch in persons who have some degree of SOK-LOONG. I have been able to corroborate this in my clinical practice and have had this demonstrated to me by Dr. Trogawa. However, Clifford miscounts the thoracic vertebrae in her work, thus placing the second point one vertebra too low.[62]

Tibetan medicine says that massage with an oil medium is very helpful in treating Wind disorders.[63] This can be a full body massage once per week or the massage of those points discussed above which are found to be sensitive to palpation. In Tibetan medicine, "medicinal" butter is considered the best medium although regular butter and vegetable oils are also acceptable. It is interesting to note the revived popularity of massage in America at a time when Tibetan medicine says we can use it all the more. The massage of individual points with butter or oil can be done on a daily basis by the patient or their family members. One patient with whom I have tried this felt he benefitted greatly from it. Epstein and Rabgay suggest that of the so-called secondary measures in the treatment of Wind psychoemotional disorders, massage with oil is especially beneficial.[64]

Tibetan dietary recommendations for Wind disorders are both interesting from the point of view of Chinese dietary therapy and more comprehensive than their Chinese counterpart. Since Wind is light and airy, foods which are considered light and airy should be avoided. These foods are the opposite of oily. they tend to be cooling and dry. Such foods include: coffee, tea, alcohol, potatoes, tomatoes, spices, goat meat and milk, sugar, refined flour products, raw vegetables, and salad greens. Dr. Trogawa simply describes airy foods as "everything which is not nutritious"[65], i.e. junk food. Also undereating or fasting can aggravate or even cause Wind disease. Therefore Tibetan medicine recommends a high protein diet emphasizing meat, soup made from bones, hot milk, whole grains, seed oils, butter, and, strangely enough, onions and garlic. Food in general should be eaten cooked and warm.

From the Chinese point of view, and the Tibetan, if the Liver is not participating in the formation of Flaring Fire due to its being Damp and Hot, oil is not contraindicated. If the Liver is, however, as is most often the case, at least in Americans according to my experience, then one must be careful with one's intake of oils. Also in such cases, more salad greens can be eaten in order to reduce the TRI-PA or Bile (Fire) of the Liver. A careful analysis of the etiology of each patient's disorder must be made in order to determine the fine points of dietary therapy. However, the above generalizations, I think, make theoretic sense in both systems and have been borne out in my clinical experience. Sufferers from Wind disorders are also usually counselled to eat several small meals per day instead of a couple of large one. Tibetan medicine literally believes that food in the gut can weigh down the up-fluttering Wind in the same way that the Chinese use Cinnabar and Dragon Bone to weigh down the fluttering SHEN.

Looking at the diets of most Americans between the ages of twenty and forty, one can identify, according to Tibetan medicine, an overconsumption of coffee, tea, alcohol, caffeinated soft-drinks and chocolate, sugar, salads, spices, and cold and raw foods. It is interesting to note that the imbalances created by these foods are often aggravated by fasting, strict vegetarianism, and raw food faddism in those proponents of "natural" healing in their efforts to rid themselves of the "toxicity" of the standard American diet. Such persons swing from one extreme to the other and in my experience only fan the flames of imbalance created in their youth. Rather than such faddism being healthy, it often leads to, in Chinese terms, Deficiency of Yin and Blood. It is often very difficult to convince such patients that a "heavier", less "pure" diet is actually in their best interest. It is as if, once we become imbalanced, it becomes very difficult to discern where true balance lies since the individual must always look through the filter or distortion of their imbalance. This goes back to the notion of our not having an imbalance but being imbalanced. In addition, the fixation on purification as the sole model for attaining good health itself belies a frenetic inability to relax and accept things as they are. It is only another symptom of our culture's neurosis.

Besides diet, it is very important that a person suffering from Wind should live in a warm, congenial atmosphere. Cold and windy environments are detrimental to persons with a Wind disorder. They should not spend too much time in direct sunlight, as in sunbathing, nor should their rooms be too bright. Rather they should be surrounded by subdued colors and lots of greenery and vegetation. Green in general is a good color for LOONG disorders and Dr. Trogawa recommends green carpets in such cases. The patient should preferably sleep on the ground floor, wear warm clothing, and have a comfortable bed which will induce and encourage sound and copious sleep. As much as possible, they should be surrounded by friendly, warm, congenial persons and they should refrain as much as possible from competition, discord, violence, and stress. Above all, as Dr. Trogawa says, they should laugh.

Such persons should not indulge in too much sensory input of any kind, for, in fact, in such cases, the nervous system simply needs to rest, to cool down. Persons should not overwork, stay up late, nor talk too much. Responsibility is a negative thing for a person with a stress-induced mental disorder. Therefore having to work under a watchful boss is contraindicated, as are deadlines and other forms of psychological pressure. All noise is contraindicated in Wind disorders, whereas quiet is indicated. This applies to background music in general and rock 'n roll in particular. Too much sex is contraindicated but too little in also not good. Wind is created at its root by Desire. Therefore a happy medium must be met between suppressing desire and overindulging it. This applies particularly to sex and in this matter Tibetan and Chinese medicine agree. According to Chinese medicine, too much sex weakens the Kidneys and exhausts the JING. This leaves the SHEN without support.

It is my belief that our modern preoccupation with sex is a direct outgrowth of our culture's general overheating. One of the symptoms of Flaring of the MING MEN HUO is hyperaphrodisia. In other words our preoccupation with sex is due to the Industrial Revolution. As our culture has become more stressful and quicker paced, our desire has "naturally" been fanned. This creates even more Heat and Deficiency of Yin. It is a great relief to live for some time in a country such as China where one can spend weeks without being sexually titilated by provocative clothing, sex-oriented advertising, or the promise of promiscuity. Returning to America one becomes aware of just how prurient our society has become.

Exercise, such as calisthenics and jogging, is good for persons who suffer from Wind disorders as long as it is not overdone. Chinese medicine holds that neurasthenia is most often encountered in persons who exercise too little and think too much. Tibetan medicine agrees but emphasizes that exercise must be moderated to fit the capabilities of the patient. If the patient is too weak, exercise is contraindicated. Too much exercise will only weaken the system further. In other words, exercise, as in frenetic activity, is not necessarily the key to good health. It is best if our physical exercise is a natural part of our lifestyle as in walking, bicycling, and laboring physically. Trying to jam a whole day's worth of exercise into a half hour is often only another form of overload.

Tibetan medicine also makes use of the inhalation of certain types of incense for the treatment of Wind disorders. There is something logical about breathing in medicine to treat a pranic or Qi disorder since the problem is associated with the breath in its larger meaning. Terry Clifford describes such incenses in TIBETAN BUDDHIST MEDICINE& PSYCHIATRY.[66] The ingredients used are all likewise ingredients in Oriental herbal medicine. I have used such Tibetan incenses for calming the mind with good results both in myself and in my patients. When first studying meditation with my Tibetan Lamas fifteen years ago, I would sometimes bring Japanese, Indian, or Chinese incenses to our meditation center. In those days, because their English was not so good, I thought their preference for Tibetan incense was only cultural chauvinism. Their explanations were restricted to simply saying that Tibetan incense was better for the mind. Now, many years later, I begin to see why it is better for the mind and for meditation than other incenses whose main aim is to smell pleasing. Such therapeutic Tibetan incenses are presently available in the United States from Blue Poppy Enterprises whose address is given in the endnotes.[67] Nutmeg powder burned on an incense charcoal is a simple substitute. It is called the King of Incense and regulates the Life-wind.[68]

Likewise, Tibetan medicine believes that breath exercises, called TSA-LOONG THIG-LE in Tibetan and QI GONG in Chinese, are particularly beneficial in the treatment of Wind disorders. This is because of the close connection between breathing and the LOONG. However, breath exercises wrongly practiced are also an easy way of developing SOK-LOONG. Therefore, it is very important that such exercises be learned from a well-practiced and experienced teacher who can diagnose the individual and teach that person just the right techniques for his or her individual imbalance. I have written at length about the merits and dangers of such exercises in BLUE POPPY QIGONG to which interested readers are referred. In that book I have especially discussed the danger signs of QI GONG-induced Wind imbalance and described those persons for whom this type of practice is unsuitable.

Terry Clifford discusses a number of Tibetan herbal medicines used for treating psychoemotional Wind disorders. I have not discussed these along with Chinese herbal treatments since their composition and use differ markedly from their Chinese counterparts. Tibetan medicine is Buddhist medicine. It is a spiritual medicine, not a materialistic medicine. Within the Tibetan herbal formulary there are a number of prescriptions which generically are called RIN-CHEN RIL-BU or Precious Pills. These formulae were usually revealed by great spiritual masters. They are most often a type of TER-MA or Hidden Treasure, a particular class of scripture or doctrine believed to be of divine source. These RIN-CHEN RIL-BU are composed not only of herbs and minerals but also of relics from great saints and sages. They are compounded as part of a ritual which mystically imbues them with divine power. Often such rituals last for days on end. The spiritual power and Realization of the officiating Lamas directly affect the potency of the pills. Therefore, RIN-CHEN RIL-BU made by some Lamas are more highly sought after than others. It is believed by Tibetan Buddhists that many of these RIN-CHEN RIL-BU have been revealed as the specific remedies for the diseases endemic in this degenerating KALI YUGA.

As Terry Clifford says, "This is a kind of spiritual supermedicine."[69] When Ms. Clifford asked H.H. Dudjom Rinpoche, the Grand Lama of the oldest or NYING-MA sect of Tibetan Buddhism, what medicine, if any, would be helpful in treating the mental illness so prevalent in our modern world, His Holiness suggested a RIN-CHEN RIL-BU called "The Precious Essence that Removes sorrow from the Mind" (SEM-KYI DUNG-SEL RIN-CHEN NYING-PO). This formula is atrributed to Yuthok Yonten Gonpo, the Hippocrates of Tibetan medicine, a famous doctor-saint who lived in the eighth century CE.

These RIN-CHEN RIL-BU are taken in very small doses. They are not even taken every day. For patients whose main complaint is not psychoemotional disturbance, they should only be taken once and a while. Tibetan medicine places great importance on the astrologocal timing of the treatment. Therefore, the 8th, 15th, and 30th days of each lunar month are considered auspicious days on which to take RIN-CHEN RIL-BU. Also the first fifteen days of the first lunar month and the first fifteen days of the fourth lunar month are particularly auspicious. Tibetan Buddhists believe that anything, good or bad, done on these days will reap a reactions one hundred thousand times more powerful than usual. the pill should be crushed and added to a Cup of pure water the night before the dose is to be taken. This should be kept out of direct light and traditionally this cup is placed on the family altar. This should then be drunk in the morning upon arising on an empty Stomach. Nothing should be eaten for at least one hour after taking the pill. If a Buddhist, the patient should say the Medicine Buddha mantra and do the appropriate visualization as taught by their Lama. For the entire day the patient should rest, refrain from talking, working, exercising, and avoid emotionally stressful situations. They should meditate quietly of possible and not eat meat, garlic, onions, spicey foods, stimulants, alcohol, or take any other medications. They should also abstain from sex. For one RIN-CHEN RIL-BU I am familiar with these proscriptions last for three weeks after taking a single pill. These proscriptions allow the medicine to affect the flow of LOONG through the psychic channels or meridians at a very subtle level.

It is my feeling that these RIN-CHEN RIL-BU work at a deeper level than Chinese herbal formulae. I also feel they are compatible with correctly prescribed Chinese formulae. In my practice, I will suspend regular Chinese prescriptions for a day or so when administering RIN-CHEN RIL-BU. The patient then resumes taking their Chinese formula the next day. I look on these pills as a way of accessing a deeper level of energy than the Chinese herbs do and as a way of affecting changes in the patient on a spiritual level.

RIN-CHEN RIL-BU are currently being made in Tibet under Red Chinese supervision. The Chinese value these pills so highly they reserve 90% of those manufactured in Lhasa for use by high government cadres in Beijing. Various types of RIN-CHEN RIL-BU are also made to treat Bile and Phlegm disorders. Some are quite effective for treating various types of "poisoning", hepatitis, certain cancers, and musculoskeletal diseases. One type is excellent for bringing a latent Evil back up to an acute manifestation for more direct treatment. I hope to write further on my experiences using these pills in future publications. Blue Poppy Enterprises markets a number of different RIN-CHEN RIL-BU here in the US which are made in Tibetan monasteries in Nepal, Sikkim, and the Indian Himalaya.

People who are really crazy usually cannot relax themselves. To suggest meditation or deep relaxation to such patients may be unrealistic. However, for the treatment of the early stages of mental disorder, which, it is my contention, most young Americans suffer from, meditation and deep relaxation are, according to Dr. Trogawa, very beneficial. This statement includes the vast majority of us ambulatory neurotics with red-tipped tongues. Although exercise helps to "bleed off" or vent rebellious or congested energy, exercise will not stop the production of Excess Wind. Meditation or deep relaxation can. As such, these are root treatments; whereas exercise is only a branch treatment. Relaxation is a skill. One's ability to relax can be trained and developed over time.

While studying in China, I visited a hospital in Shanghai which had a ward devoted to the treatment of stress-related disorders with meditation/deep relaxation. Although the doctors referred to their treatments as QI GONG, what they demonstrated to me were various standing and sitting versions of traditional Buddhist and Taoist meditation. These doctors had accumulated voluminous data which led them to make certain statements on the requirements of therapeutically effective deep relaxation. Statistically significant changes in blood chemistry, Galvanic Skin Response, brain waves, blood pressure, and temperature in the extremities, all in a more positive and healthful direction, can be obtained if the following criteria are met: 1) that the relaxation technique results in physical or muscular relaxation as well as mental equipoise; 2) that the center of consciousness be lowered subjectively from the head to below the waist; 3) that the technique be practiced continuously from twenty to thirty minutes per day; and 4) that the technique be practiced every day without missing a single day for a minimum of six weeks.

There are many types of meditation/deep relaxation available here in the United States. Not all of these meet the therapeutic requirements outlined above. For the average patient, I usually recommend any one of the commercially available relaxation tapes as the easiest and cheapest way to fill the above "prescription". However, Tibetan medicine does have additional suggestions regarding the therapeutic employment of relaxation as part of a treatment plan for correcting a Wind disorder. The following pieces of advice are based on the oral instructions of the Ven, Dr. Trogawa Rinpoche.

If possible one should find a grassy hill or knoll on which to sit with the slope falling away from one leaving an expanse of space in front. Nothing should block one's vision. One should sit and look out across this space and think about nothing, i.e. as soon as one becomes aware that th are engaged in thinking they should let the thought process relax and dissolve itself. The breath should be light, long, and stressing the exhalation with a light aspiration sound. It is best to do this practice at sunrise and sunset. In the morning face the West. In the evening face the East. In other words, sit with one's back to the sun. If one finds themself near a river, stand or sit and watch the water flowing away to sea identifying their thoughts and problems with the ever-flowing quality of the stream.

In BLUE POPPY QIGONG I have discussed the benefits of meditation/deep relaxation more fully and have given a more elaborate meditation technique based on Tibetan yoga which combines the requirements of the above-mentioned Chinese research with Dr. Trogawa's advice. Michael Broffman has also suggested that patients with red-tipped tongues should sit and relax on the shaddy banks of streams or in other "Yin" environments such as cathedrals. Biofeedback and Hatha yoga corpse pose are also excellent, therapeutically beneficial ways to fill this prescription. However, one must be careful, since the wrong meditation can, in fact, cause meditation-induced SOK-LOONG.[71] Any meditation which causes internal pressure, stress, frustration, and a raising of the center of consciousness, for instance to the tip of the nose, will tend to create a Wind imbalance or aggravate an existing one as one of the appended case histories wil show. Many spiritual practices intentionally try to induce an aggrandisement of the Wind humor. In a carefully monitored practice under the guidance of a well-qualified and experienced spiritual master this is a natural part of the spiritual path. However, for the general public working without expert guidance this can be dangerous.

In the West we like to talk about and analyse our psychoemotional problems. In fact, we have created in the space of eighty years at least half a dozen professions whose job it is to help us analyse and "deal with" our neuroses. For the most part, Oriental medicine, whether Tibetan, Chinese, or Japanese, does not encourage this and I also personally think most psychotherapy for the average neurotic is counterproductive. Our neuroses are the product of our minds just as are all and every mental events, whether they be rational thoughts or irrational feelings and emotions. Thinking about thoughts is a never-ending loop. Trying to change one set of thoughts by another is like squeezing quicksilver. Thinking about our neuroses, talking about them, trying to analyse them or cathart them, all add fuel to their fire. The fundamental problem is that the mind is racing out of control. Because it is overheated and stressed, it produces unhealthy, imbalanced thought and emotions. If the mind is simply allowed to rest in peace, it will naturally and spontaneously begin to produce a happier, healthier product. This belief in the intrinsic sanity and health of the nature of the mind is the foundation of all traditional Oriental psychoemotional "therapies".

In his excellent book on Japanese "psychotherapy", THE QUIET THERAPIES: JAPANESE PATHWAYS TO PERSONAL GROWTH, David Reynolds describes the racing mind as one in which the spacing between thoughts is jammed too closely together. "The functioning of the disturbed person's mind has been mispaced. Either it has been unchecked, fleeing from topic to topic to escape distressing thoughts and feelings, or it becomes stuck on some obsessive rumination or in some compulsive ritual. All of the quiet therapies effect this pacing of the flow of thought by isolating the client, reducing the stimulus input available to his senses, and encouraging him to be physically still. The result is a slowing of thought processes and, it is believed, a deepening of them as well."[72] Reynolds continues: "A premise underlying these simple therapeutic strategies is the fundamental Buddhist one that man is essentially good ... Quiet isolation brings about the opportunity for our natural inner strength to lead us toward a more enlightened understanding of ourselves."[73]

It is my experience that talking about, analysing, and attempting to cathart neuroses never really change or cure the individual. Such activities often only teach the patient how to be more skillfully neurotic by using a more erudite vocabulary to rationalize their behavior and short-comings. Oriental medicine suggests that emotional outbursts only further exhaust and deplete the individual causing more Flaring of Deficiency Fire in the Heart. Perhaps if a patient's energy is blocked by stifled anger, one skillfully managed catharsis may set the stage for the beginning of the healing process. But repeated pillow-beating, weeping and wailing, and other currently popular forms of emotional self-indulgence are, in the long run, energetically counterproductive. Ultimately the root of the problem is the erroneous belief in the independent existence of the individual ego. Therapies which focus their attention on this ego, thus validating it, only serve to reinforce the root of the problem. As Ms. Clifford writes, "Mental and emotional strain cause the winds or airs to increase. Thinking and concentrating on something too much, worrying about unfinished projects and unattained goals, grieving over family troubles, and becoming upset over lost articles -- all these are said to disturb the wind and thus the mind, since the wind and the mind are bound together."[74]

American patients do not come to the practitioner of Chinese medicine seeking treatment for Flaring of Deficient Heart Fire. They do come for insomnia, anxiety, palpitations, chronic sore throats, skin rashes, menorrhagia and metrorrhagia, cystitis, vaginitis, chronic herpes, spermatorrhea and premature ejaculation, cataracts, tinnitus, vertigo, rheumatoid arthritis, Lupus, ulcers, hypertension, and chest pain. Without exception, every patient that I have seen and treated for the above problems in the last five years has exhibited a red-tipped tongue. A detailed description of the mechanisms involved in the production of these symptoms vis a vis Deficient Fire is beyond the scope of this work. The knowledgable practitioner should, however, be able to figure out the mechanisms of each of these symptoms using the theories of Traditional Chinese Medicine. Nor do I have the leisure to give a detailed treatment plan for each of the above. What I am suggesting is that Deficiency Fire be given a great deal of thought in the diagnosis and treatment of twentieth century Americans. And I am also suggesting that treatment beyond the symptomatic level aiming at prevention should utilize other therapies beyond just acupuncture and herbs.

Ultimately, the only true treatment of flaring of Deficiency Fire in the Heart is a spiritual treatment. The root cause of this problem is our belief in a false ego and our desire to bolster and protect it. In this endeavor, we separate ourselves from the source of life, willfully attempting to go against the greater flow and eventually burning ourselves out in this attempt. According to Tibetan medicine, each of the humors is correlated with one of the Three Poisons, the three aberrations of the egoistic mind which cause it to suffer. LOONG or Wind is created and supported by fire of desire, lust, or attachment. It is this fire of desire which manifests as Ministerial Fire on the mundane level. Rather than Heat, the Fire of the Kidneys should be transformed into Light at the Heart, the Light of Enlightenment. This alchemical transformation into Light is part of the nature of reality. It is a process which has its own intrinsic rules and laws and in order to ourselves participate in this transformation, we must consciously recognize and live by these laws.

Although this dilemma seems to be reaching epidemic proportions, not to mention catacylismic, this is the ancient existential dilemma as expressed in the following famous dialogue between the Yellow Emperor and his doctor, Chi Po. "The Yellow Emperor asked: 'I have heard that ancient people were able to live to one hundred years and still be the same as when young. But nowadays, when fifty years old our activities decrease. How is this? Is it due to the times, or have humans lost something?' The physician Chi Po answered: ' The ancients knew the Way, the Tao, and the rule of Yin and Yang. They lived in harmony with numbers (i.e. they lived by natural law as expressed in numerology and astrology). The ancients controlled their eating habits. They knew the rules of life, waking and sitting. They didn't overwork. Thus they were healthy and balanced in body and mind and were able to live to one hundred years. But today, people are not like this. They drink too much alcohol and think about sex. After drinking they go to bed and lose their JING according to their desire. At the same time as losing their JING, they lose and disperse the truth. They don't know how to control their mind and cannot control their desires. They are against the living pleasure, the Tao.'"[75]

Chi Po does not really answer Huang Ti's second question as to whether this degeneration is due to the cycles of time. Buddhist medicine suggests our present degeneracy is due to the pervasive influences of the KALI YUGA. Still, each of us as individuals has the freedom to recognize this degeneracy and to correct it in ourselves. Oriental medicine, both Tibetan and Chinese, gives us the tools to see and correct this degeneracy in terms of our health. Buddhism gives us the key to unlock the problem of our ego at its fundamental root.

CASE HISTORIES

The first two case histories presented below relate to meditation related or induced neurasthenia. In classical Chinese medicine there is a class of disease called CHAN BING or meditation disease. Although meditation/relaxation is perhaps the single most important corrective for stress-induced disorders, faulty meditation can, in fact, aggravate or cause these same disorders.

A thirty-nine year old man had had extreme fatigue, tidal fevers, insomnia, hypertension, night sweats, dizziness, tinnitus, polyuria, and nocturia for several months. His western MD had diagnosed his disorders as psychosomatic and stress-induced. He had prescribed Inderol, a beta-blocker. The patient had taken Inderol for some time and this had alleviated his palpitations. However, the patient did not want to take allopathic drugs. As soon as he discontinued the Inderol, the palpitations returned and his other symptoms worsened. Upon my examination I observed a red-tipped, tender, slightly fluted, and quivering tongue with scant white fur. His pulse was thready and rapid, especially for such a large, seemingly vigorous man. On palpating his abdomen, I found an abnormally strong pulse in the descending aorta. This patient was balding and had smallish ears with very thin helixes. My diagnosis was Yin and Qi Deficiency with Flaring of Heart Fire.

This man's problems had begun when, after reading some books on spiritual pursuits, he and his wife went to Thailand to become a Buddhist monk and nun. for a number of months they meditated intensively using the so-called New Burman SATTIPATTHANA technique. This technique uses as its "support" concentration on the tip of the nose. Husband and wife lived in separate compounds and both maintained strict celibacy. The diet was purely vegetarian and completely Thai. Speaking of this particular meditative technique, Mahathera Sangharakshita says: "... investigation revealed, however, that it (this method) was not without its dangers. As taught by some teachers, at least, and as practiced by some pupils, it could lead to extreme nervous tension and to a schizoid state ... On my return to England in 1964 I met twelve or fourteen people who were suffering from severe mental disturbance as a direct result of practicing the so-called 'VIPASSANA Meditation'."[76] Zhou Da-heng, in THE CHINESE EXERCISE BOOK, explains one reason for the ill effects of this technique based on clinical experimentation in China: "It has also been demonstrated that blood pressure drops when attention is focused on the lower abdomen, while it rises when attention is focused on the tip of the nose."[77] In this patient's case, the lack of protein to which his body was unaccustomed, the strain of celibacy for a married man, and both the forced intensity and poor choice of meditative technique were compounded by a severe case of dysentery which further exhausted his Yin.

After several months, both the patient and his wife became disillusioned with their teachers and their monastic life. They returned to the United States where the man tried to continue his meditation practice while at the same time experimenting with various extreme yogic and "detoxifying" practices. He ate only raw fruits and vegetables, fasted frequently, and did different types of purges. Mentally he also suffered from guilt due to the warning by the Thai monks that by leaving the monastery he would "burn in Hell". This guilt was compounded by his loss of self-esteem due to his inability to work in his weakened condition thus throwing the burden of their financial support entirely upon his wife. When he came to see me the slightest exercise or exertion would completely exhaust him for several days. Even eating caused him to feel nauseous and feverish and to break into a sweat.

I explained to the patient his diagnosis from both the traditional Chinese and the Tibetan medical perspectives. He was very relieved to finally understand what in fact was happening to him. At that time, although I was familiar with Tibetan medical theory, I had had very little experience with its therapeutic modalities and did not have access to any Tibetan RIN-CHEN RIL-BU. Therefore although I counselled him to stop his meditation practice, to eat animal protein, to refrain from drinking too much water, and to eat nourishing, cooked food, all from a Tibetan perspective, I chose to treat this patient with a contemporary TCM approach for SHEN JING.

I prescribed GEJIE DA BU WAN patent medicine as an herbal medication to consolidate his Kidney Qi, tonify Kidney and Liver Yin, and to tonify Qi and Blood, including the WEI QI to stop the spontaneous and night sweating. His acupuncture treatment consisted of needling SAN YIN JIAO (Sp 6), TAI CHONG (Liv 3), TAI XI (Ki 3), ZU SAN LI (St 36), GUAN YUAN (CV 4), SHEN SHU (Bl 23), AN MIAN, SHEN MEN (Ht 7), NEI GUAN (Per 6), YIN TANG, and BAI HUI (GV 20). Not all these points were used every treatment. Usually I selected eight points per treatment depending upon his presenting complaints. He received from one to three treatments per week for almost three months. In this time his urination decreased, the night and spontaneous sweating was eliminated, and his digestion improved. However, most of his other symptoms persisted to some degree or came and went depending upon stress and fatigue. Even after three months of treatment, slight exercise would fatigue the patient for several days.

The patient became impatient with the slow course of treatment. He had not really learned that it was his style or approach to life and his treatment which ultimately was the cause of his problems. Finally the patient declined further Oriental medical treatment and went back on Inderol. Over one year later, the patient was still on Inderol and if he dropped his dosage below a certain level his symptoms returned.

Although this is the most extreme case of meditation-induced SOK-LOONG I have seen to date, still my opinion is that the TCM protocols I employed in treating this patient were not subtle or sophisticated enough to effectively treat this man. Although his impatience and desire to meddle with his treatment plan were a symptom of his disease, still I feel a more comprehensive treatment would have elicited more marked improvement and therefore have won his allegiance to the therapy.

A little over one year later, a man twenty-five years old came to me with a chronic sore throat and extreme fatigue. He also was a Buddhist meditator. He was tall and lean with small, highly set ears with very fine helixes. He had an angular face with a high forehead -- all signs of a constitutional predisposition to LOONG imbalance. His sore throat was worse in the morning upon arising and in the evening with fatigue. Also his ears and cheeks became red in the evening or when fatigued. His pulse was largish and slippery but empty and both CHIH positions were deepish and weak. His left pulse was markedly finer than the right. The patient's tongue had a bright red tip, slight fluting on the forward edge, and had a greasey yellow coat. The patient had been doing extreme numbers of prostrations per day in an effort to meet a certain liturgical deadline. These prostrations are extremely fatiguing physically if done too quickly or in excess and also their attendant concentration can be too tight if forced. In any case, the correct emotional tone when doing these prostrations is not a hurry-up sweat to finish by a certain day as if completing a term-paper. The patient had also had three episodes of mononucleosis since adolescence. Western allopathic examination failed to detect a recurrence of mono. His allopathic doctor suspected infection by the Epstein-Barre virus.

My intial diagnosis was Kidney Lung Yin Deficiency complicated by Phlegm Dampness. I performed acupuncture at LIE QUE (Lu 7) and ZHAO HAI (Ki 6) with gold needles and slanting the needle distally at LIE QUE. I also needled ZHONG WAN (CV 12) and FENG LONG (St 40) with stainless steel needles and deep insertion. I this case I chose to duplicate the acupuncture treatment with the following herbal formulae given in decoction:

Bulbus lilii	10 grams
Ophiopogon	10
Treated Pinellia	5
Oryza sattiva	5
Codonopsis	5
Polygonati	5
Zizyphus sattiva	3
Treated Licorice	2
Peony	5
Tang Kuei	5
Platycodon	3
Fritillaria	3

After four days the patient reported marked improvement in both his energy and sore throat. In addition he was sleeping much better, However, the herbs had made him very flatulent. Therefore I switched him to the following formula:

Codonopsis	3 grams
Poria	3
Coix	5
Dioscorea	2

Cardomom	2 grams
Atractylodes	3
Lotus Seed	4
Platycodon	2
Licorice	1.5

After a several days of taking this formula, the patient felt "almost 100% better". However, when he returned to doing prostrations or any physical exercise his symptoms and weakness also returned. I continued needling him at LIE QUE and ZHAO HAI approximately once per week and switched him to CHIH PAI PA WEI WAN for slow, steady tonification. I explained to the patient the Tibetan concept of SOK-LOONG and the TCM concept of Yin Deficiency neurasthenia. After taking the CHIH PAI PA WEI WAN continuously for one month, the patient developed Rehmannia-induced loose stools due to the complication of Phlegm Dampness in his condition. Therefore I immediately took him off this formula but then was in a quandry what to do. Most Yin tonifying ingredients tend to aggravate Dampness due to their greasey nature. It is possible to create a non-greasey Yin tonifying formula using Loranthus parasiticus and Tribulus, etc. However I did not want to give him a decoction since my experience has been that herbs for this condition must be taken over a very extended period of time and decoctions tend to be time-consuming and relatively expensive. Instead I taught him how to inhale nutmeg incense, massage with oil the Tibetan LOONG points, and to also indirectly moxa these and GAO HUANG SHU once or twice a week. The patient felt an immediate positive response to these self-administered therapies. Still, however, he had the tendency to slip back into his Deficiency weakness and feverish feeling if he overexerted himself. I then prescribed a RIN-CHEN RIL-BU for LOONG imbalance resulting in nervous disorders. He took one pill per week for three weeks on the New Moon, First Quarter (the 8th), and the Full Moon (the 15th). The patient felt that these pills helped him to finally turn the corner on his condition. In general, I use these pills to create movement in patients whose treatment has become stuck.

Seven months after initially consulting me, his ears hardly ever turned red anymore, which was for me a sign that his Yin had regenerated itself somewhat. A Doctor Wu from San Francisco, while visiting Boulder, gave the patient a further consultation. He likewise felt that the patient's digestion was too weak to digest Kidney-tonifying herbs. Instead he taught the patient some QI GONG exercises and reaffirmed the longterm importance of the patient's diet. A year later the patient still has a constitutional tendency to Flaring of Deficient Fire, which, in all probability, he will have his entire life. However he has returned to doing prostrations, albeit with a different attitude and approach. Two other interesting notes on this patient's case were that listening to loud rock 'n roll or seeing an intensely dramatic movie would worsen this patient's condition when it was still quite pronounced, and that he had a disinclination to sitting meditation since internally he was so restless.

Meditation-induced or aggravated Yin Deficiency with Flaring Heart Fire is relatively common in American communities with large populations of young people interested in alternative life-styles. As discussed above, our culture predisposes us to this disorder and our American hubris of "doing our own thing" often leads us, like the first patient described, to concoct false Dharmas based on our own willfullness. That erroneous meditation leads to Yin Deficiency with flaring of Heart Fire is exemplified by a Chinese saying regarding this phenomenon: HUO SHUO SHAO LIN SSU, or, "The fire burns the Shaolin Temple". As Kenneth Cohen explains in an article on the dangers and contraindications for QI GONG: "The fire is the heat of excessive concentration. The Shaolin, literally 'the little forest', symbolizes the hair. Thus the expression is interpreted, 'One sign of excessive concentration is that the hair follicles are burned out. One starts to lose the hair or develop bald patches.'"[78] Practitioners of Chinese medicine recognize baldness as a sign of Yin/Blood Deficiency.

The third case history describes a case of neurasthenia not related to meditation but only to neurosis. The patient was a thirty-two year old man. His major complaints were anxiety, palpitations, chest pains and tightness, dizziness, low back stiffness, knee soreness, occasional chronic sore throat, phobias of various sorts, epididymitis, various skin irrtiations, restless sleep, and cold hands when nervous or after eating. The patient reported that in the morning between 8 and 11 AM he would usually conceive a negative or hypochondrical idea which he would then compulsively worry about and depressed over. By Noon he was able to let this compulsion go although this pattern would recur the next day. The patient's stools had a tendency to be loose and these symptoms had persisted for two and a half years. During that time the palpitations had become less frequent and less pronounced.

Upon my examination his tongue was fluted and swollen, had a dry coat, was cracked in the center, and had a red tip. On presentation there was considerable trembling of the tongue. His pulse was superficial and inflated of the right, especially at the GUAN position. On the left, the pulse was threadier and the CHIH position was deep and weak. Prior to my seeing this patient, he had been to a Chinese medical clinic in San Francisco and been diagnosed as suffering from Kidney Yin and Spleen Deficiency with Deficiency Heat disturbing the SHEN. This likewise was my diagnosis.

The doctor in San Francisco had prescribed an herbal formula to be taken in decoction. Its ingredients were:

Tang Kuei	6 grams
Peony	9
Poria	6
Orange Peel	3
Ophiopogon	9
Zizyphus spinosa	9
Polygala	9
Zizyphus sattiva	3 pieces
Treated Licorice	3 grams
Polygonati	12

He was advised to take this formula and to concurrently receive acupuncture on a regular basis. Since the patient did not live in San Francisco, he was not able to follow this advice and therefore the doctor had alternatively told him to seek out a local practitioner of Chinese medicine.

Before beginning treatment with me, the patient next went to an MD who had trained in acupuncture for six months in Beijing. This doctor's diagnosis was also the same. He was only an acupuncturist and therefore his treatment plan consisted of needling SAN YIN JIAO, TAI XI, TAI CHONG, SHEN MEN, NEI GUAN, SHAN ZHONG, and ZHONG WAN. This formula is a predictable contemporary TCM acupuncture treatment plan for Yin Deficiency neurasthenia. The patient received three treatments per week for two weeks, two treatments per week for another two weeks, and received one treatment per week for several weeks on a seemingly on-going basis. The patient felt relaxed after each treatment but did not notice any cumulative effect or diminishment of his symptoms. The acupuncturist had suggested "Zen-type" meditation as an adjunctive therapy. However, the patient was unable to merely witness his thoughts without becoming involved in them and this ultimately only caused him more anxiety.

Although my diagnosis was essentially the same as the two previous practitioners', my treatment plan was not. I decided that bulk herbs in decoction were a waste of time and money since, in my experience, we were not going to achieve speedy results in any case. It takes energy to make energy. Kidney Yin is only replaced very slowly until a certain threshold of energy is reached. Strong doses of herbs in such cases are not necessarily better or more effective. Instead I suggested that the patient take GUI PI WAN, a patent medicine in pill form, for slow and steady and affordable tonification. Next, I suggested that he not receive the formulaistic type of acupuncture he had been. I did not feel that such acupuncture was going to achieve speedy results either, and in fact, it had not. The most important thing that I have found in managing such cases is the necessity of the patient's understanding the cause and nature of their imbalance. This implies that the success of the treatment relies on the patient's modifying their life-style. It also implies that the patient must take a longterm view of their situation and not look impatiently for a quick fix.

Therefore I further outlined the dietary recommendations to reduce Deficiency Heat, tonify the Kidneys, and to tonify the Stomach/Spleen. This included eating more animal protein since the patient had been attempting a raw foods vegetarian diet based on its being more "healthy" and "spiritual". I suggested that he rub oil onto his upper torso daily and also inhale nutmeg incense on a regular basis. I prescribed for him a RIN-CHEN RIL-BU for LOONG imbalance to be taken once per week for three weeks. I taught the patient a relaxation technique using breath awareness and concentration on his lower abdomen. This technique gave him something definite to do and gave him a sense of mental steadiness which the other meditation had not. I suggested that he get a job instead of sitting around all day and especially recommended a job doing gardening or light physical labor for the summer with no managerial responsibiltiy. And finally, I suggested that he see some funny movies, avoid intense dramatic or suspenseful entertainment, and to try to have sex once a week but to avoid masturbation.

All these various guidelines and their explanations gave the patient a sense that I really understood his problem and that I was in control of his situation. In this case I encouraged a certain amount of transference. I endeavored to be kind and supportive while at the same time confident and authoritative. After taking the GUI PI WAN for a week and one RIN-CHEN RIL-BU, the patient reported less chilling in his hands and a genral sense of improvement. After two more weeks on GUI PI WAN, his stools were consistently firm and his digestions was quite good. Therefore I switched him to TIAN WANG BU XIN

TAN and CHIH PAI PA WEI WAN for longterm use. After one month his epididymitis was gone and his palpitations were infrequent. Three months later all the patient's symptoms had been alleviated and the patient felt confident and optimistic about his life and future. Again this patient will have to be careful the rest of his life, but now he knows and understands what will cause his condition to slip backwards and the responsibility for his health is in his own hands.

Based on the above cases and a number of similar ones I have seen over the last several years, I have come to the conclusion that treatment for Yin Deficiency neurasthenia should be light and subtle and sustained. As an intern in Shanghai, I saw many such cases caused by the excesses of the Cultural Revolution. Their treatment by acupuncture was essentially the same as that tried by the practitioner mentioned above who had studied in Beijing. Eight to ten points were needled three times per week for months on end. Treatment continued either *ad infinitum* or was aborted due to frustration. I can categorically state that I never saw a case of Yin Deficiency neurasthenia successfully and conclusively treated with acupuncture during my study in China. Acupuncture treatment for such problems needs to be minimal and precise, and herbal treatment should likewise stress low dosages over long periods of time. And, what can not be repeated too often, successful cure depends primarily on the patient's life-style modification. Since Yin Deficiency with Flaring of Fire in Heart also corresponds to what some modern physicians refer to as "time disease", the keywords for everyone involved are to make haste slowly.

ENDNOTES

1 Ma Chien-chung, "Methods of Tongue Diagnosis", OHAI Bulletin, LA, Vol. 6, #1, 1981, p. 13

2 Ibid., p. 13

3 Yang Chih-yi, "Tongue Diagnosis", OHAI Bulletin, Vol. 6, #1, 1981, p. 30

4 Pao Tien-pai, "Tongue Diagnosis", OHAI Bulletin, Vol. 6, #1, 1981, p. 49

5 Anon. Committee, ACUPUNCTURE: A COMPREHENSIVE TEXT, Shanghai College of Traditional Chinese Medicine, John O'Connor & Dan Bensky, trans. & ed., Eastland Press, Chicago, 1981, p. 23

6 Ibid., p. 54

7 Porkert, Manfred, THE ESSENTIALS OF CHINESE DIAGNOSIS, Chinese Medicine Publications Ltd., Zurich, 1983, p. 136

8 Kaptchuk, Ted, THE WEB THAT HAS NO WEAVER, Congdon & Weed, NY, 1983, p. 150-1

9 Ibid., p. 54

10 Yang, op. cit., p. 31

11 Porkert, op. cit., p. 141

12 Kaptchuk, op. cit., p. 71

13 Ibid., p. 54

14 NAN CHING, study materials of the O.I.C.S.A.A. Master of Acupuncture Program, Miami, 1979, p. 98

15 Ibid., p. 99

16 Porkert, op. cit., p. 69

17 Ibid., p. 69

18 Anon. Committee, COMMON TERMS OF TRADITIONAL CHINESE MEDICINE IN ENGLISH, Beijing Medical College, Beijing, 1980, p. 20

19 Chang Hsien-cheh, "The Concept of Pathology in Chinese Medicine After the Sung Dynasty", OHAI Bulletin, LA, Vol. 9, #7, 1984, p. 337

20 Lu, Henry C., GRADUATE COURSE IN ADVANCED CHINESE MEDICAL PHILOSOPHY, Chinese Foundations of Natural Health, Vancouver, p. 6

21 Matsumoto, Kiko & Birch, Stephen, FIVE ELEMENTS AND TEN STEMS, Paradigm Publications, Higganum, CT, 1983, p. 69 & 121

22 Matsumoto, Kiko, etymological discussion in a seminar in Boulder, CO, Winter, 1985

23 Lu, op. cit., p. 7

24 Skinner, Stephen, THE LIVING EARTH MANUAL OF FENG SHUI, Routledge & Kegan Paul,London, Boston, etc., 1982, p. 37

25 Chace, Charles, lecture on abdominal palpation, Boulder, Summer, 1984

26 Lu, op. cit., p. 7

27 Chang, op. cit., p. 338

28 COMMON TERMS OF TCM, op. cit., p. 434

29 Ibid., p. 438

30 Lu, op. cit., p. 7

31 Chang, op. cit., p. 338

32 Sung Hyoun Baek, Oriental Medical Research Inc., Chicago, class notes on the Chinese pharmacopeia, 1981

33 Trogawa Rinpoche, Amche Lama Semphel, lecture, Boulder, Fall, 1984

34 Norbu, Namkhai, INTRODUCTION TO TIBETAN MEDICINE, Shang Shung Edizioni, 1982, p. 9

35 Clifford, Terry, TIBETAN BUDDHIST MEDICINE & PSYCHIATRY:THE DIAMOND HEALING, Samuel Weiser Inc., York Beach, ME, 1984, p. 132

36 Ibid., p. 132

37 Ibid., p. 132

38 Ibid., p. 132

39 Donden, Yeshi, Introductory Lectures on Tibetan Medicine, xeroxed reprint of lecture notes given at the University of Virginia, Spring, 1980, p. 20

40 Clifford, op. cit., p. 132

41 Epstein, Mark & Rabgay, Lobsang, "Mind and Mental Disorders in Tibetan Medicine", TIBETAN MEDICINE, Dharamsala, India, Series #5, 1982, p. 74

42 Bramlett, Rusty, lecture notes on the acupuncture treatment of psychological

disorders given at the New England School of Acupuncture, Boston, 1983, in turn based on lectures attended by Mr. Bramlett at the Nanjing College of Traditional chinese Medicine, Nanjing, PRC

43 Lecture notes from International Acupuncture Training, Shanghai College of Traditional Chinese Medicine, Shanghai, PRC, Spring, 1983

44 Broffman, Michael, lecture notes from Third Annual Rocky Mountain Healing Arts Festival, Summer, 1979

45 Epstein & Rabgay, op. cit., p. 75-6

46 Kaptchuk, lecture notes, Denver, CO, Summer, 1984

47 ACUPUNCTURE: A COMPREHENSIVE TEXT, op. cit., p. 626

48 Norbu, op. cit., p. 10

49 Allione, Tsultrim, WOMEN OF WISDOM, Routledge & Kegan Paul, London, Boston, etc., 1984, p. 198

50 In Tibetan, the word for skill is THABS. It implies taking a negative situation and somehow turning it to one's advantage.

51 Mann, Felix, THE TREATMENT OF DISEASE BY ACUPUNCTURE, William Heinemann Medical Books Ltd., London, 1980, p. 53

52 Kaptchuk, lecture notes, Denver, CO, Summer, 1984

53 Lu Gwei-djen & Needham, Joseph, CELESTIAL LANCETS, Cambridge University Press, Cambridge, London, etc., 1980, p. 78

54 Ibid., p. 178

55 Woolerton, Henry & McLean, Colleen J., ACUPUNCTURE ENERGY IN HEALTH & DISEASE, Thorsons Publishers Ltd., Wellingborough, UK, 1979. p. 31

56 Lecture notes, Shanghai Coll. of TCM, Spring, 1983

57 Matsumoto, Kiko, lecture notes, Boulder, Winter 1985

58 Woolerton & McLean, op. cit., p. 57

59 Yang Ji-zhou, ZHEN JIU DA CHENG (THE GREAT COMPENDIUM OF ACUPUNCTURE & MOXABUSTION), excerpts trans. by Charles Chace appearing in this volume, "The Eight Extra Meridians: Their Clinical Use According to the ZHEN JIU DA CHENG"

60 Norbu, Namkhai, lecture notes on Tibetan moxabustion, Conway, MA, Fall, 1983

61 Norbu, Namkhai, ME-TSAI LAK-LEN SHAY-GYI ME-LONG, xeroxed reprint of handwritten ms. in Tibetan

62 Clifford, op. cit., 140

63 Ibid., p. 142-3

64 Epstein & Rabgay, op. cit., p. 79

65 Trogawa Rinpoche, lecture notes, Boulder, Fall, 1984

66 Clifford, op. cit., p. 143

67 Blue Poppy Enterprises 2140 Pine St. Boulder, CO 80302

68 Clifford, op. cit., p. 207

69 Ibid., p. 200

70 Tibetan Medical Institute Newsletter, Dharamsala, India, Dec. 1982, p. 11

71 Epstein & Rabgay, op. cit., p. 77-8

72 Reynolds, David K., THE QUIET THERAPIES: JAPANESE PATHWAYS TO PERSONAL GROWTH, University Press of Hawaii, Honolulu, 1982, p. 103

73 Ibid., p. 104

74 Clifford, op. cit., p. 139

75 Based on a translation by Kiko Matsumoto appearing in THE FIVE ELEMENTS & TEN STEMS, op. cit., p. xi

76 Sangharakshita, A SURVEY OF BUDDHISM, Shambhala, Boulder, 1980, p. xv

77 Zhou Da-hong, THE CHINESE EXERCISE BOOK, Hartley & Marks, Washington, DC, 1984, p. 123

78 Cohen, Kenneth, "Chi Kung, The Danger Signals", CHI POWER, INSIDE KUNG-FU, Burbank, CA, May 1985, p. 83

TIBETAN MOXABUSTION

An Introduction for American Acupuncturists

During the Cultural Revolution, the Red Guard sacked Tibet. Iconoclastic youths destroyed the temples, monasteries, statues, and religious libraries which Tibetans had taken twelve centuries to create. This devastation and cultural genocide left few exceptions since the Tibetan culture is completely founded upon and permeated by the practice of Buddhism, a doctrine anathema to the materialistic humanism of the Communist dictatorship. One exception, however, was the medical lore of Tibet. Although much of this was also destroyed, still there was the recognition that Tibet's rich heritage of medical knowledge and experience could be of great benefit to the masses of China. Tibetan medicines are distributed to cadres and high officials in Beijing.[1] A pharmocopeia of Tibetan medicinal herbs was printed in Chinese in Qinghai in the early '70s before the fall of the Gang of Four.[2] A traditional Tibetan hospital has reopened in Lhasa. I have seen copies of the GYUD ZHI, the preeminent classic of Tibetan medicine analogous to the NEI JING, preserved in the library of the Shanghai College of Traditional Chinese Medicine and own a copy of a recent Chinese translation sold in that college's bookstore.[3] I have also purchased copies of a Tibetan medical dictionary and the biography of Yuthok Yonten Gonpo, the patron saint of Tibetan medicine, recently reprinted and sold at the Xin Hua Shudian in Shanghai. As His Holiness the Dalai Lama has said, "In fact, because of its usefulness, despite the Chinese's deliberate destruction of Tibetan culture, they have left the Tibetan medical system intact and have even preserved and promoted it."[4]

Although some Chinese medical researchers are obviously interested in the arcane knowledge of Tibetan medicine in China today, there is the tendency in general clinical practice to simplify what is called Traditional Chinese Medicine to a point which disturbs many classicists such as myself. An ultra-simple and I believe simplistic form of acupuncture, as characterized in A BAREFOOT DOCTOR'S MANUAL, gained ascendency in Chinese clinics during the 60s and 70s. During this period, many of the surviving old masters of Chinese medicine were forced into retirement after being "criticized", i.e. beaten, whether physically or mentally, for their adherence to "reactionary superstition". It is unfortunately still fashionable to dismiss many of the more subtle insights and techniques developed during the Song, Yuan, and Ming dynasties as clinically unverifiable mumbo-jumbo. Doctors in contemporary Chinese clinics pay so much attention to the major complaint that the systemic imbalance is often overlooked. And all too often, little or no attention is paid to prevention. Many of these trends have likewise influenced the training in and practice of Chinese medicine in the United States. Traditional Chinese Medicine or TCM forms the basis for the curriculum of several American acupuncture schools such as the New England School of Acupuncture and the American College of Traditional Chinese Medicine. However, as one of my colleagues puts it, TCM is not so much true traditional Chinese medicine as it is WTDICT, What They Do In China Today.

We live in a basically materialistic and humanistic time. Modern culture is fundamentally secular. True classical Chinese medicine was cosmological as opposed to egocentric, energetic as opposed to materialistic, and spiritual as opposed to secular. The great names of Chinese medicine were all intensely spiritual men such as Zhang Zhung-jing, Ge Hung, Sun Si-miao, Tao Hung-jing, Liu Wan-su, and Zhu Dan-xi. It is my belief that most of our modern problems, whether individual, societal, or environmental, are due to the degenerate trend towards materialism, secularism, and egocentricity. The chronic, recalcitrant diseases running rampant in our society today, such as cancer, diabetes, heart disease, and auto-immune disease, are due to this same degeneracy. Modern medicine, which includes contemporary TCM, since it is a product of the times, is likewise following this same downward spiral. This has led to the growing inability of modern medicine to provide sound care which the public trusts and believes in. This also accounts for the proliferation of iatrogenic disease.

However, using the same heteropathic logic which is the foundation of Chinese medicine, if a disease is due to creeping materialism, then it should be offset or balanced by a more "spiritual" approach to medical treatment. This essay is a presentation of Tibetan moxabustion lore and practice. It is offered in the possibility that some of its esoteric, cosmological insights might prove useful to modern clinicians seeking to treat the decadent diseases of this time. Although Tibetan and Chinese medicine are not identical, it is my belief that some of the practices kept alive in Tibetan medicine can be applied to Chinese medicine in order to redress some of the oversimplification of Chinese medicine which has occured in the recent past.

The material in this essay is largely based on Namkhai Norbu Rinpoche's Tibetan language book on moxabustion entitled ME-TSAI LAK-LEN SHAY-GYI ME-LONG (THE CRYSTAL MIRROR OF THE PRACTICE OF MOXABUSTION).[5] This has been supplemented by Namkhai Norbu's oral commentary on his text given in Conway, Massachusetts in the Fall of 1983 and on lectures given by the the Ven. Dr. Trogawa Rinpoche in Boulder, Colorado in the Fall of 1984.

Moxabustion is one of the five modes of treatment covered in the fourth or last volume of the GYUD ZHI (THE FOUR MEDICAL TANTRAS). These five modalities are bloodletting, moxabustion, inhalation of medicinal vapors, the wearing of mineral substances next to the body, and medical salves and massage. The section on moxa is divided into seven subsections. These are: 1) the collection and preparation of the moxa wool; 2) indications; 3) contraindications; 4) principle points for the application of moxa; 5) methods of application; 6) post-treatment closure; and 7) the benefits of moxa therapy.

The preparation of the moxa should be performed by the doctor himself for best effect. This is because the energy of the doctor will effect the material being prepared. In Tibetan medicine the doctor is usually a religious person who has undergone intensive spiritual development. Just yeaterday a Tibetan doctor intending to visit the United States wrote to ask when we collect our herbs and I was chagrined to think of his perplexity when I have to inform him that most American practitioners rely on store-bought ingredients. The spiritual development of the practitioner and the practitioner's psychic effect on both the medicaments and the patient are points completely overlooked in modern TCM. The herb, Artemesia vulgaris sinensis, should be gathered during the three autumn months. In a warm country or climate it should be gathered during the first month of autumn, i.e. late August. In a cold country it should be collected during the last month. The element associated with the day of the week and the constellation, i.e. the 28 lunar mansions of Oriental astrology, should be harmonious and should promote the Fire element. For instance, Sunday and Tuesday are related to Fire. Wednesday, however, is related to Water which adversely controls Fire. Therefore Wednesday is not considered a propitious day for the collection of moxa. The entire area the herb is to be gathered from should be purified by sprinkling with consecrated water at the same time the doctor performs a purification visualization and mantra. This is to remove the DUK or toxins associated with the herb due to the surrounding geomantic energy. The herb this then pounded a bit in the wet state in oder to make it "stronger". It is next dried in the shade. After it is dried, it is rubbed to remove the stems and other impurities, all the time repeating a mantra such as the Medicine Buddha's. Finally a small bit of charcoal made from soft wood is mixed into the Artemesia wool.

According to Tibetan medicine, the indications for moxabustion are Internal Deficiency of Heat, as in digestive deficiency problems, water accumulation problems, various types of stones, such as kidney, gall, etc., all kinds of lymphatic disturbances, nervous and psychoemotional problems, certain types of Phlegm disorders, and many types of traumatic injury. Moxa is deemed excellent for meridian obstruction problems and for "closing" a point after bloodletting. Moxa is contraindicated, however, immediately after giving birth, just after diarrhea, before bloodletting, or when the nerves and channels have been cut and stitched back together. It is also contraindicated in the treatment of most, but not all, febrile diseases and for blood circulation problems such as hypertension. Also moxa is contraindicated on certain points at certain astrological times.

This last contraindication deserves further discussion. Tibetan medicine possits the existence of several LA-NAY. The LA is the vital energy of the individual, family, or country. The LA-NAY is the place where this vital energy is thought to reside or concentrates. It is the place where the Spirit attaches to the matter. This is not a single, static point in the human but several points which move through the body in relation to certain astrological cycles each of which relates to a different aspect of the person's life-force. Therefore there is a LA-NAY for the year, day of the lunar month, day of the week, and the hour of the day. Any trauma striking one of these LA-NAY will have a disproportionate effect on the life energy of the person. As a person dies, the LA comes apart from the body and disease becomes irreversible if the LA deteriorates past a certain point. Likewise the point of the LA-NAY can have a profound negative effect on the cure of a serious chronic disease if that point is harmed through heroic treatment. Namkhai Norbu, quoting an ancient Tibetan text on astrology, says, "When we have the LA connected with the life-force (SOG-LA), if at these points blood is drawn or moxa is burned, this could even kill an ill person. And if these methods are used on points where the LA connects with the physical body, the person can get infected or get a types of nervous disorder in which the nerves and muscles in the area will not function properly. If one does moxa or bloodletting at the WANG-THANG (the place of personal power), this may diminish the power or the capacity of the individual. If at the LUNG-TA (the "Wind Horse" or place of personal fortune), these therapies can lessen the length of life. If at the KYE-LHA(the site of the good spirit associated with birth somewhat akin to the western concept of the guardian angel), these can damage the physical power of the individual."[6]

The place of the LA-NAY can be calculated with the aid of an astrological almanac. Both the Chinese and the Tibetans share essentially the same astrological and calendrical systems. Determining the LA-NAY is somewhat analogous to finding the "open" points according to the ZI WU LIU CHU LIAO FA, the Chinese astrological system of determining which of the 66 Antique points are most accessible to acupuncture at any given moment in time. Since much Tibetan moxabustion is direct moxabustion with scarring and since such a heroic treatment may harm the LA, such measures must not be applied to the site at which the LA is concentrated.

Below are the positions of the LA-NAY according to Namkhai Norbu and modified by Trogawa Rinpoche. In some cases it is not clinically convenient to find a time when a certain point is totally safe from proximity to any of the several LA-NAY. Of the four LA-NAY calculable, it is most important and easiest to avoid the LA-NAY for the hour of the day. Secondly, the LA-NAY for the year is easy to remember and important. The LA-NAY for the day of the week and the day of the lunar month are less important.

The LA-NAY for the year correlated with the BA GUA, called BAR-KA in Tibetan. These are the eight primary trigrams of the I JING or BOOK OF CHANGE. According to Namkhai Norbu, these are numbered one through eight, although, since these are also correlated with the numbers one through nine of the so-called Magic Square, this may be a simplification in terminology for western students not versed in the intricacies of Oriental astrology. One is related to the trigram LI or Fire. Two is related to the trigram KUN or Earth. Three is related to TUI or Lake. Four is related to QIAN or Heaven. Five is related to KAN or Water. Six is related to GEN or Mountain. Seven is related to SUN or Wind. And eight is related to CHEN or Thunder. I have used the Chinese names since these are the ones with which most readers will be familiar. Even the Tibetan names are merely obvious transliterations of the Chinese. They are in order: LI, KHON, DVA, KHEN, KHAM, GIN, ZIN, and ZON. According to Namkhai Norbu, 1983 was associated with trigram number eight, CHEN/ZON. Therefore, 1984 was associated with trigram one, LI and 1985 is associated with trigram two, KUN/KHON. Since Namkhai Norbu mentioned that 1983 was the last year in the sixty year cycle, I am assuming that the trigram changes at what even in Tibet is sometimes referred to as Chinese New Years. However, according to Shao Yung's system of Chinese astrology which predates the introduction of the Chinese calendar into Tibet, the trigrams change at the winter solstice and not at Chinese New Year.[7] Each trigram is associated with a particular part of the body. During the year ruled by a particular trigram, moxabustion is contraindicated on points on that body part. The chart below summarizes these correspondences.

LI	Head
KUN	Left hand & arm
TUI	Left torso
QIAN	Left leg & foot
KAN	Reproductive organs
GEN	Right leg & foot
SUN	Right torso
CHEN	Right arm & hand

The LA-NAY for the day of the week is calculated as follows:

Sunday the LA resides in the Head	
Monday	Chest
Tuesday	Lungs & Liver
Wednesday	Waist
Thursday	Hips & lumbar region
Friday	Kidneys & spinal vertebrae
Saturday	Bladder

The LA-NAY associated with the day of the lunar month starts its progression on the first day from the soles of the feet and travels according to the following cycle:

First	Soles of feet
Second	Lower legs
Third	Thighs
Fourth	Waist
Fifth	Inside of mouth
Sixth	Palms of the hands
Seventh	Ankles
Eighth	Elbows
Nineth	Reproductive organs
Tenth	Waist
Eleventh	Ears
Twelfth	Forehead
Thirteenth	Teeth
Fourteenth	Heart
Fifteenth (Full Moon)	Crown of head
Sixteenth	Sternum
Seventeenth	Throat
Eighteenth	Stomach & insides of thighs
Nineteenth	Thighs
Twentieth	Face
Twenty-first	Soles of feet

Twenty-second	Hips
Twenty-third	Lower legs
Twenty-fourth	Palms of the hands
Twenty-fifth	Tongue
Twenty-sixth	Neck
Twenty-seventh	Shoulders
Twenty-eighth	Reproductive organs
Twenty-nineth	Pupils of the eyes
Thirtieth (New Moon)	Disperses throughout the body

When I had occasion to show Trogawa Rinpoche these placements for the daily LA-NAY, he suggested that they were generally correct but were not quite exact enough for really accurate location.

And finally, the LA-NAY for the hour of the day is located using the Chinese 120 minute "hour" or the twelve Terrestial Branches. Therefore there are twelve Chinese hours in a day and twelve different locations for the LA-NAY each twenty-four western hours.

6 AM	Feet & legs
8 AM	Neck & mouth
10 AM	Lips
Noon	Chest & eyes
2 PM	Navel & tongue
4 PM	Heart
6 PM	Spinal column
8 PM	Feet
10 PM	Sex organs
Midnight	Stomach & sex organs
2 AM	Chest & solar plexus
4 AM	Intestines

The reader familiar with Chinese astrology and with Chinese acupuncture will note that Namkhai Norbu lists the hours beginning at our Midnight and Noon, i.e. 12 PM and 12 AM. Although I cannot say for sure this is not the traditional Tibetan method of reckoning the hours of the day, in Chinese astrology ZI is likewise often translated as Midnight but as a time period it begins at our eleven PM not at twelve. It is my guess that Norbu Rinpoche did not take into account this fact. Therefore it is my suggestion that this progression should begin at five AM not six. This corresponds more accurately with the twelve Terrestial Branches as usually applied to the hours of the day. The reader will also note that some Tibetan astrologers reckon the day beginning at sunrise, not at Midnight, as Norbu Rinpoche has done here.

Moxa will also prove to be an ineffective treatment in general during several other astrological periods. The first two are the ZHI-SHE and the DUN-ZUR. The ZHI-SHE are the fourth year before and after the patient's year of birth as calculated by the twelve Terrestial Branches. For example, if a person is born in a Tiger year, moxa will be an ineffective treatment for this person throughout either the year of the Snake or the year of the Pig. The DUN-ZUR is the seventh year ahead of the year of birth. In this case, moxa will be ineffective for a Tiger person in any Monkey year.

Likewise there are certain times which are ruled by spirits whose nature is Watery and therefore moxa, a Fire treatment, is not effective during these times. There are two such times called BISHTI and LU RIK-DEN. These are calculated as follows: Afternoons in general are the time of the BISHTI on the fourth, eleventh, eighteenth, and twenty-fifth days of the lunar month. Mornings are not propitious for moxa due to the influence of the BISHTI on the eighth, fifteenth, twenty-second, and twenty-seventh. The times of the LU RIK-DEN are Sundays from 10-11 AM, 11 PM - Midnight, and 4-6 AM; Mondays from 7-8 AM, 2-4 PM, and 2-4 AM; Tuesdays from Noon - 2 PM, 2-4 PM, 8-10 PM, and 2-4 AM; Wednesdays from 8-10 AM, Noon - 2PM, and Midnight; Thursdays from 10 AM - 1 PM and from 10 PM - 2 AM; Fridays from 9 AM - Noon and 9 PM; and Saturdays from 6-10 AM and from 8 PM - Midnight. The reader should note once again that based on the way these times are presented, Namkhai Norbu is following the tradition that the new day begins at dawn. Therefore it is still Sunday until 6 AM of what we would call Monday morning. The LU RIK-DEN are very powerful Naga spirits or snake/dragon spirits associated with underground water, lakes, rivers, oceans, and rain. Since Water controls Fire, moxa administered during the hours of the LU RIK-DEN will not be very hot.

Tibetan medicine, although it speaks at length of the TSA or channels, has not ennumerated and catalogued points in the same way as Chinese medicine. Rather than learning a list of points on a channel, the Tibetan doctor-to-be learns the list of points which are appropriate for moxabustion. He also learns a list of points for acupuncture, bloodletting, cupping, and massage. Points on these lists may overlap but often they do not. In other words, a point may only be a "moxa point" or an "acupuncture point".

According to the Tibetan system of classifying points appropriate for moxabustion, there are two types of moxa points: 1) what the Chinese would call AH SI or locus dolendi points, points where pain or the symptoms of a disease are directly located; and 2) points indicated in the treatment of a disease distant from the site of the symptoms and derived from principle and experience. In a text by Yuthok Yonten Gonpo, 60 principal moxa points are discussed. Namkhai Norbu discusses 360 moxabustion points. These are based on his research of ancient Tibetan and Zhang Zhung medical texts while in Beijing in the summer of 1983. These are grouped according to body part. In his text there are 99 points on the back of the torso, 70 points on the front, 72 points on the head, 58 points on the upper extremities, and 62 points on the lower extremities. However, since most of these points are bilateral, the Chinese enumeration of them would be a little more than half this number.

From my observation of Dr. Trogawa Rinpoche, it seems that Tibetan doctors are much more precise in their location of moxa points than the majority of their Chinese counterparts. There are three types of measurement used for locating points. The first is called TSUN. It is equal to the width of the thumb joint. The word TSUN is obviously borrowed from the Chinese word CUN (寸). A CHAK, which means hand in Tibetan, is the width of all five fingers including the thumb. A CHI is the equivalent to the width of seven fingers. Tibetan doctors are careful to always use the patient's hand as the standard of measurement and cut sections of dried grass twigs to precisely measure out the location of the points. Since a great deal of moxabustion in Tibetan medicine is burned directly on the skin leaving a scar, erroneous location of a point may not only diminish the effectiveness of the treatment but will also leave a sign of the practitioner's lack of skill to be read by succeeding physicians. Ballpark location is not acceptable. This precision, I believe, has its merits.

There are four ways which moxabustion is actually applied to the body. The first is called TSO-WA which means to cook. This is the repeated burning of large cones of moxa directly on the skin. It is the strongest and most heroic moxa treatment in Tibetan medicine and is used for cancer and other types of tumors. TSO-WA is for more serious conditions and can be repeated up to 20 times. SEK-PA means to burn. It is the second method of application. Here the moxa is allowed to burn down to the skin but is them immediately removed. SEK-PA is for the treatment of Phlegm disorders, lymphatic problems, and certain nervous disease called NI-LUNG in Tibetan. It can be repeated up to fifteen times. These two methods must be performed by a professionally trained physician and calculation of the LA-NAY is important.

SO-WA means to heat. This is an indirect moxa treatment using a moxa roll similar to Chinese moxa rolls, which, however, Tibetan doctors feel are inferior to the Lama-doctor prepared ones. The point is heated just until a small blister is raised. SO-WA treats nervous disorders, diseases due to Kidney weakness, and the malfunction of certain channels. DIK-PA means to slowly transmit heat to an area without raising a blister. It is used when treating children, the weak, and the chronically ill. Both SO-WA and DIK-PA are used when the disease is not violent or acute. If a disease is acute with more violent symptoms, the first two methods are usually used.

Tibetan medicine also pays close attention to the "closure" of the points after moxa treatment. If TSO-WA and SEK-PA have been used, the physician is directed to massage the points with his thumb. Then the patient is asked to take a short walk. The patient is advised not to drink for a while after moxa treatment since Water negates Fire. This proscription against drinking anything Cold extends into the evening as well. Cold drinks, according to Tibetan medicine, include wine, fermented milk, and yogurt. It is also important that the patient does not do any strenuous activity which would make him or her sweat. And, for one week after treatment, the patient should not nap in the middle of the day. All these post treatment proscriptions are designed to maximize the effectiveness of the treatment.

According to Tibetan medicine, the benefits of moxa are several. It regulates the functions of the channels. It eliminates pain. It treats diseases provoked by LOONG or Wind, one of the three humors of Tibetan medicine. LOONG diseases can affect any part of the body, but in America it is most important to note that LOONG diseases are often caused by emotional stress. Most nerve disorders are due to a LOONG imbalance. Moxa controls various types of swelling, dries up edematous areas, and eliminates pain in the chest caused by the accumulation of Phlegm. Moxa treats such diseases as cancer, ulcers, and old wounds. It regulates and harmonizes the functioning of the internal organs and increases the Fire of life. It clears the mind and it cures diseases which are otherwise resistent to other forms of treatment.

Of the peculiarities of the Tibetan use of moxabustion discussed so far, I particulary think American practitioners of Chinese medicine could benefit from considering the following: First, the preparation of the moxa by the physician himself. Moxa, or Artemesia vulgaris, does grow wild in many parts of the

United States. Local gathering and preparation takes advantage of the local geomantic influences and potentizes the moxa with spiritual Qi through the conscious processing of the practitioner. Although this cannot be quantified or measured by materialistic science, Kirlian, photographs, lie detectors, and other somewhat objective "proofs" suggest that, in fact, one's conscious intent does have an impact on vegetable and inorganic substances.

Secondly, the contraindications based on Oriental astrology are, I believe, important. If one is doing direct moxabustion with large cones of moxa, following such astrological rules will minimize the possibility of infection according to Trogawa Rinpoche. Although direct moxa is not popular in America, it is very effective according to Tibetan doctors in treating tumors and cancer. Also, by following these astrological guidelines, one can maximize the positive effects of a treatment by using the macrocosmic flow of energy to support the microcosmic flow in the patient. This conscious employment of timing adds a dimension of sophistication to the treatment which can reduce the total number of treatments a patient must receive. It also promotes a more holistic attitude in the practitioner as a servant of the macrocosm which in turn can empower the practitioner to be a more potent healing force himself. And finally, it teaches forebearance, patience, and attention, all of which are positive qualities in a human being let alone in a healthcare provider.

Third, as mentioned above, I believe the more precise location of points using paper, string, twigs, or a ruler also helps to sharpen the precision of the practitioner's intervention. This too maximizes the effect of the treatment with a consequent reduction in the needed number of office visits and again minimizes the likelihood of infection. Since acupoints have a higher concentration of Righteous energy, they are more resistant to infection. Likewise this care and attention to detail helps to calm the mind of the practitioner. When the practitioner's mind becomes relaxed and clear, he or she can be a more effective healer from both a rational and suprarational point of view. This means the practitioner cannot be running from treatment cubicle to treatment cubicle or rushing from one patient to the next. Such care and attention to detail also increases the confidence of the patient in the competency of the practitioner which is also of great therapeutic benefit.

Fourth, post treatment closure and behavior proscriptions are very helpful in maximizing all the positive benefits of the treatment. They allow the patient to participate more fully in the treatment and to continue the treatment after leaving the clinic. Personally I often feel the Qi moving in my body for at least a day, and often for several, after receiving moxa treatment. Walking after a treatment helps to promote the free and easy flow of energy generated and liberated by the moxa. The gentle circulating effect of walking will help the Qi seek its own level like running water.

And fifth, as Tibetan medicine suggests, moxa should be investigated as a potent adjunctive therapy in the treatment of cancer. Acupuncture is often too late to do anything more than relieve pain in many cancer cases. Moxa, especially direct moxa, is a more powerful treatment combining the effects of acupoint stimulation, heat, and the herbal properties of Moving Stagnation inherent in Artemesia vulgaris. When a person's life is at stake, scarring due to moxa treatment should not be a great concern. Likewise moxabustion offers economical and effective treatment for the many nervous disorders which beset modern man and for which modern medicine either can only say, "It's all in your head", or drug the person into oblivion, neither of which approaches being very beneficial.

Many modern acupuncturists are reluctant to use moxa since it is "smelly", "dirty", and "time-consuming". It does not fit in well in a sanitized, antiseptic, expensively decorated clinic. This reluctance is all part of our cultural decadence, our superficiality, and the artificiality of our lifestyle. I have had a patient die because the hospital in which he was would not allow him to moxa himself because of the smell even though the treatment had shown signs of improving the patient's condition. In old China, many doctors specialized entirely in moxa, such as Ge Hung's wife,[8] and there is an entire classic devoted to it, the HUANG TI MING TANG MOXA CLASSIC. Tibetan medicine suggests we likewise should not just think of moxa as a dispensible adjunct to acupuncture but that American practitioners should accord moxa the status it rightly deserves. After all, the Chinese ZHEN JIU, which is often simply translated as acupuncture, means acupuncture <u>and</u> moxabustion.

In addition to the above five benefits from studying Tibetan moxabustion practice, a look at the names and indications of some of the Tibetan "moxa points" which are identical in location to recognized Chinese acupoints may, in some cases, add a fresh perspective on the use and nature of these points. Not all Tibetan moxa points are identical to Chinese acupoints but below are a number of points important to both systems where, I believe, the Tibetan literature has something quite useful to add or to underline.

DA ZHUI (GV 14) is called LOONG-SANG or the Wind point. When treating with moxa, the tip of the vertebral prominence itself is warmed. This point in Tibetan moxa literature is used to treat all nervous, neurotic, and psychic disorders due to LOONG or Wind. This is the Tibetan concept of Wind which actually is closer to the Chinese concept of Qi than to Wind as a pathological Excess. Symptoms include trembling, aphasia, palpitations, daytime somnolence, insomnia, certain types of headaches associated with the Wind, and a grey or whitish tongue.

The Bladder Associated points on the back are very similar in general in the Tibetan system to the Chinese. One difference is that at each vertebral segment there are three points all of which bear the same name. There are the two points on either side of the vertebra and a third point on the midline itself at the tip of the spinous process. This point on the midline is considered the principal point and the side points are used as auxilliary points in more severe cases. Actually the side points correspond to the HUA TO JIA JI points, not the Bladder Shu points since they are located only one TSUN lateral to the midline, not 1.5. However their energetic nature is similar. For the most part the indications and organ ascriptions are the same as in Chinese. The following, however, bear special mention.

SOG-TSAI SANG, the Life Channel point(s): These correspond to JUE YIN SHU (Bl 14). The Life Channel carries a subtle Wind or Qi intimately associated with the Heart and the Mind. If an inappropriate energy enters this channel and displaces the Life Wind, various nervous system symptoms will appear. The person may become crazy or agitated. The body may tremble or shake. There may be lack of self-control, amnesia, and goose-bumps all over the body. The head may feel heavy or congested. There may also be water retention around the Heart due to worry. This is called SOG-LOONG for short in Tibetan and basically means the person is mentally unbalanced.

In the Chinese system this point is not named for an organ as are the majority of the Shu points, although in English it is called the Pericardium Associated point. It is named for a level of energy, the JUE YIN, which is intimately connected with the Heart, the Liver, and the MING MEN HUO. This point is used in Chinese medicine to regulate the function of the Heart, as in the treatment of Chest BI syndrome or angina pectoris. The Tibetan usage and nomenclature for this point suggest a more profound usage emphasizing the psychoemotional balance and integration of the individual, on the one hand, and their SOG or life-force on the other. This larger meaning has numerous implications concerning the relationship between the Liver and the XIN BAO (Pericardium), the XIN BAO and the MING MEN HUO, and the connection between the Kidney Fire and the Heart and the JING and the SHEN. Pondering these implications could even affect how a Chinese style acupuncturist might chose to use a JUE YIN channel point such as NEI GUAN (Per 6).

THRI-PA SANG means the point of the Bile. Bile is one of the three humors of Tibetan medicine. This point corresponds to DAN SHU (Bl 19), the back Associated point of the Gallbladder in Chinese medicine. Although it is indicated in the treatment of jaundice and gallstones, moxabustion at this point is also suggested for the treatment of poor eyesight, headache due to Bile, and runny nose due to insufficient Heat in the Stomach. In general, since the Liver/Gallbladder tend to be Excess according to Chinese medicine, many Chinese style practitioners do not think of moxaing this point. However, looking at the above Tibetan indications, I would suggest trying moxabustion on this point for the treatment of upper respiratory allergies to animal hair, a symptom usually associated with Dampness in the Middle and Deficiency Heat in the Liver.

Bladder 22 and the point at the tip of the lower edge of the spinous process of the first lumbar vertebra are called the first KAY-TSHIG points. KAY-TSHIG means lumbar vertebra in Tibetan. In the Tibetan system these points are associated with the TSAM-TSE which means the Gate of Life. This is the Tibetan translation of MING MEN. In the Chinese system, Bladder 22 is called SAN JIAO SHU or the Triple Heater Associated point. It is seldom encountered in modern clinical practice since the Triple Heater is not seen as a separate organ and therefore "it" cannot be disordered. Any so-called imbalances of the Triple Heater are more accurately described by the interrelationship of the organs and bowels which make up the Triple Heater. Therefore in Chinese one can talk about an Upper Heater imbalance which is shorthand for a Lung/Heart pattern of disharmony.

In the Tibetan system, by relating these points to the MING MEN HUO, as opposed to Governing Vessel 4 as in Chinese acupuncture, a clearer clinical picture of this point's applicability emerges. According to Namkhai Norbu, it is used in treating either men or women with lack of control over discharges from their sexual organs. In men this would correspond to spermatorrhea. In women this relates to Kidney Deficiency leukorrhea. It is also good for treating uterine "stones" or tumors, extreme dysmenorrhea (probably due to Cold), and dry feces (due to Kidney Deficiency).

SHEN SHU (Bl 23) is also called the Kidney point in Tibetan. However, this also includes Governing Vessel 4 as explained above. It treats Kidney Deficiency problems of various sorts. In addition, it treats Large Intestine problems which underscores the close relationship between the Kidneys and the Intestines through the so-called Internal Duct of the Triple Heater. This is a connection largely overlooked in modern TCM. Also, Tibetan texts suggest that moxa on this point can help ensure the birth of a male baby in a woman who habitually gives birth to girls.

QI HAI SHU (Bl 24) is called the point of the Organs and Bowels. Interestingly, the Tibetan system cautions the practitioner not to moxa this point on the right side as this will cause eye disease. The left side controls procreative energy and in the Tibetan system the point is mostly used to treat infertility. In the modern Chinese system it is only used to treat low back pain. However, in bestowing a name like the Sea of Qi, the ancients must have had more significant uses for this point which, it seems, the Tibetan Lama-doctors have retained. By naming this point the point of the Organs and Bowels, I believe the Tibetans have underscored the relation of the Pre Natal Qi to the Post Natal functioning of the organism somewhat akin to Zhang Jing-yue's theory of the seventeenth century.

BAI HUAN SHU (Bl 30) is called the Anus point in Tibetan. BAI HUAN means white circle in Chinese. When I was a student of acupuncture I asked several Chinese doctors what this white circle was. None could tell me until one doctor in Shanghai looked it up in a classical text and informed me that the white circle was a reference to the smooth white shincter muscles around the anus. The Tibetan name confirms this. Moxa at this point relieves waves of pain in the area, i.e. tenesmus, as well as all types of anal pain.

SHAN ZHONG (CV 17) is called NYING-SANG CHEN-MO in Tibetan. This means the Great Mother of the Heart point. Moxa here is indicated for the treatment of palpitations, a sensation of emptiness in the region, great sadness, and an inability to eat (due to emotional distress). If one does eat, they cannot digest their food.

TE-WAI SANG, the Navel point, corresponds to SHEN QUE (CV 8) in the Chinese system. It is particularly used for gynecological problems. It regulates the menses, treats LOONG or Wind problems after childbirth, difficulty in conception, and habitual miscarriage. It is flanked by LONG-GI DUN-SANG corresponding to TAIN SHU (St 25) with similar usage as in Chinese medicine and further lateral by LONG-PHUK SANG corresponding to DA HENG (Sp 15).

On the head, YANG BAI (GB 14), TAI YANG, and YIN TANG all have corresponding Tibetan moxabustion points. YANG BAI is called MIK-SANG which means Eye point. It can be moxaed for dry eyes with no liquid, eye fatigue, and for eye disease in general. YIN TANG is called MIN-SANG or Eyebrow point. It treats MIK-SER or yellow eyes due to jaundice, eye weakness due to Bile, and uncontrollable epistaxis. TAI YANG is called MIG-ZUR SANG. Moxabustion at it is indicated in Tibetan medicine for the treatment of inflammation of the eyes, loss of memory, loss of or poor coordination, and loss of consciousness.

JIAO SUN (TH 20) is called NA-WAI LHEN-SANG which means On Top of the

Ear point. This point is classically forbidden to needles in Chinese medicine. It has an effect on the body's biological clock and it helps to regulate the aging process. Namkhai Norbu's moxa text, however, does not recognize these subtleties in the use of this point. Rather, the sole indication he gives for moxaing this point is the treatment of torticollis. Although this is a somewhat mundane use in comparison, it is an interesting addition to the Chinese indications.

REN ZHONG (GV 26) is called CHU-GONG SANG, Above the Lip point. It is moxaed for difficulty speaking and for blurting out words without meaning. Enough said.

FENG CHI (GB 20), an important and commonly used point in Chinese acupuncture, is not very important in Tibetan moxabustion. It is called CHU-WAI SANG, Trapezius point, and it is moxaed for neck rigidity and headaches. Head WAN GU (GB 12), on the othe rhand, is not an important Chinese acupoint but does have more Tibetan indications. It is used for headache, sleepiness, and lack of presence. Both these points are not commonly moxaed in TCM since most Gallbladder related problems manifesting symptomology in the head tend to be Excess and Yang. It is interesting to note that the Tibetans do nor seem to fear the exacerbation of such problems by the use of moxa. Care, however, must be exercised in patients suffering from hypertension.

LIE QUE (Lu 7) is called THEB-RU SANG in Tibetan. Moxa at this point treats fevers from influenza, lingering fevers, eye illnesses, a burning sensation in the eyes, and opthalmia.

QU CHI (LI 11) is called SHU-KYOK SANG in Tibetan. Moxa at this point benefits the production of the fluid which lubricates the joints and benefits the functioning of all the joints.

LA-SUL SANG is the Tibetan name for FENG SHI (GB 31). It is moxaed for sciatica of the leg and foot, for pain which "boils up", and for difficulty walking or sitting.

QU QUAN (Liv 8) is called CHU-GYU SANG. Moxabustion here according to Tibetan texts regulates the menses and treats menorrhagia.

YANG LING QUAN (GB 34) is called KANG-DONG SANG. It is also used to regulate the menstrual cycle and to treat amenorrhea. No mention is made of using this point for joint and locomotive problems as in Chinese acupuncture. Its use as a gynecological point is also different from its usual Chinese usage.

DU BI (St 35) is called LHANG-OK SANG which means Crow's Eyes point. It is often moxaed in Tibetan medicine. In Chinese medicine this point is used only to treat knee pain. In Tibetan medicine it is used for improving the digestion, reinforcing the eyesight, and only third for pain in the leg.

ZU SAN LI (St 36) is also commonly used in Tibetan moxabustion practice. It is called CHU-SER SHONG-SANG. However, from Namkhai Norbu's description, it seems only to be used for problems of the lower leg. It is moxaed for pain in the bones of the leg, throbbing pain in the leg, muscle cramps, and all illnesses below the knee.

YONG QUAN (Ki 1) is called KANG-THIL SANG in Tibetan. It is moxaed to treat lymph diseases, various foot problems, and all types of eye problems.

Many Tibetan moxa points are not identical to Chinese acupoints. Some of these may be useful additions as Extra points to the Chinese style clinician. Unfortunately, since their location requires more space than this essay can devote, I will only give two such points as examples. One is called THEB-SANG or Big Toe point. It is located on the top of the big toe in the middle of the knuckle crease. Moxa on this point treats insanity, loss of the faculty of reason, mutism, paralysis due to stroke affecting the movement of the head, and orchitis. The second point is called MIG-GI RING-SANG or the Distant point of the Eyes. It is on the back of the heel where the achilles tendon attaches to the calcaneous. Moxa on this point benefits the eyes, treats opthalmia, treats madness, nervousness, and internal pressure, and is also indicated in the treatment of all disorders provoked by possession.

Although Chinese and Tibetan medicine are not identical, they are close cousins. Certain Tibetan medical traditions assert that their use of acupuncture and moxabustion clearly came originally from China. If that is so, and I believe all the evidence points in that direction, then these therapies entered Tibetan culture most probably during the Tang, Song , Jin, and Yuan dynasties. After that time Tibetan culture turned in upon itself and fostered its own self-imposed isolation. It is therefore my belief that Tibetan medicine keeps alive a more holistic and subtle medical tradition than modern TCM. It is also my belief that practitioners of Traditional Chinese Medicine could learn much of value from studying Tibetan medicine without necessarily abandoning their own system or devoting the twelve years traditionallyrequired to become a Tibetan doctor. Chinese medicine is, in general, easier to learn, easier to administer, and is perhaps more culturally and climatically suited for use in America. However, certain techniques and insights of Tibetan medicine may help Chinese style practitioners deal more effectively with those aspects of disease and treatment relating to timing. i.e . astrology, spiritual and demonic influences, psychological imbalances, and tumors and cancers. The following case history documents my experience using Tibetan moxabustion technique in the treatment of a type of psychoemotioal imbalance that Chinese medicine sees but poorly.

The patient was a woman in her mid thirties. Several years prior she had suffered what her western doctors considered a mild stroke. She had lost consciousness and fell to the floor. She lay there paralysed unable to get to the phone. As she reflected upon her situation it seemed clear to her that no one would come to her aid for at least several days. For some reason the patient believed that most fatalities from stroke occur when the patient does not receive life-support quickly and therefore she assured herself that she was going to die. Based on this conviction or fear she then went through all the psychoemotional stages associated with dying such as anger, grief, and resignation. These finally culminated in an out of body and a spiritual peak experience.

The patient was found and she did not die. It took her a year to overcome her paralysis and to be able to speak without an apoplectic slur. After her experience she was a different person. Her previous relation to herself and her life had collapsed. She left her job and friends and moved back to Kansas to be near her family as she tried to create a new reason for living and a new lifestyle. However, her family and friends in Kansas also lacked a conceptual framework to account for this woman's seemingly irrational behavior.

This woman regularly had feelings of energy rising up through her body and into her head. This caused her great pain but often great bliss as well. She felt as if the energy were forcing open unused portions of her brain. She felt energy coursing through her body. When this energy was blocked she experienced pain. If this energy moved through the blockage, she felt more integrated, powerful, and at ease. This woman also experienced visions, prophetic dreams, and other parapsychological phenomena. The only place she was able to find a support group in her area was at a local Tai Chi class. Her instructor recognized that this person was experiencing some kind of spontaneous spiritual process. He taught her various Qigong exercises, some of which helped her and some of which aggravated her symptoms. Feeling that he did not have enough training in dealing with such a situation he referred this woman to me.

Her Tai Chi instructor thought that acupuncture might fascitate the energetic process that seemed to be unfolding with difficulty. She came to see me and it became apparent that she had two levels of imbalance manifesting simultaneously. On one level she suffered from PMS due to Liver Qi Congestion. This manifested as premenstrual emotional lability and depression, constipation, sore breasts, and menstrual irregularity. Her pulse was wirey and her tongue was reddish purple with a thin yellow coat. On a deeper level, the patient was experiencing a spontaneous arousal of Kundalini about which she was uninformed and for which she was unprepared. This premature loosening of the Kundalini was due to the opening of all the bodymind's normal gates and locks during the death process. Like many people who have entered the death process and then returned to their bodies, all these gates and locks had not fully closed.

On the level of Liver Qi Congestion causing premenstrual tension, Chinese herbal medicine and dietary therapy are quite effective. For this I prescribed JIA WEI XIAO YAO WAN[9] and suggested the patient not eat too much greasey, spicey food, too much red meat, too much difficult to digest food such as nuts and refined flour products, or any coffee or alcohol. On a deeper level, the level of her being a "Kundalini casualty", modern TCM does not have an adequate diagnostic model to explain and develop a treatment plan which would take into account both the cause and the full scope of the symptoms. Esoteric styles of Buddhist and Taoist Chinese medicine may have such descriptions, but these are not currently available in English in the West. However, this patient's problems on this deeper level seemed to me to be well described as a LOONG imbalance from the Tibetan medical point of view. Therefore I decided to try some Tibetan moxabustion to treat this deeper level.

After explaining my thoughts on her case, we determined an astrologically propitious date and time to administer the moxabustion. On that day I moxaed with SO-WA technique LOONG-SANG, SOG-TSAI SANG, and NYING-SANG CHEN-MO. In addition I performed the "Golden needle" technique on the point called TSHANG-PAI GO-SANG, the Aperture of Brahma, which corresponds to BAI HUI (GV 20) in Chinese acupuncture. This technique is similar to Chinese WEN ZHEN or Warm Needle technique where moxa is burned on the handle of a gold needle inserted perpendicularly into this point. During this part of the treatment the patient could feel all the congestion in her head open up capillary bed by capillary bed. Afterwards she felt that her normally poor vision had become crystal clear and remained so the rest of that day. For several days after she did not experience the negative pains in her body or her head.

I administered this same treatment two more times in the next ten days, always at auspicious astrological times. Each time the patient reported a clearing of her head and sensorioum and a very mentally peaceful and clear next several days. After the patient returned to Kansas, she wrote to say her PMS was much better after two months of taking the Chinese herbs. I counselled her that she needed to seek out a spiritual master who could guide her through the process of unfoldment and awakening her karma had seemingly thrown her unprepared into the midst of. Six months later a young man came to see me from Kansas on the basis of the great positive changes which had occured in this woman and which were obvious to all around her. For me, this case confirmed that Tibetan moxabustion as described above can be successfully blended with contemporary TCM treatment.

ENDNOTES

[1] Anon., "Tsothay and Precious Pills", TIBETAN MEDICAL INSTITUTE NEWSLETTER, Dharamsala, India, Dec. 1982, p. 11

[2] QING ZANG GAO YUAN YAO WU TU JIAN (A PICTORAL HANDBOOK OF QINGHAI-TIBETAN PLATEAU HERBS), by committee, Qinghai Province Botanical Research Institute & Tong Ren District Long Wu Clinic, Qinghai People's Press, Xining, 1972

[3] SI BU YI DIAN (THE FOUR PART MEDICAL COLLECTION), trans. by committee, People's Health Press, Beijing, 1983

[4] His Holiness, the IVXth Dalai Lama, quoted in an advertisement for Dr. Yeshe Donden's INTRODUCTION TO TIBETAN MEDICINE and presumably abstracted from the Preface to this forthcoming book. The brochure in which this quote appeared was published by Snow Lion Publications, Ithaca, Ny, Feb. 1985.

[5] Norbu, Namkhai, ME-TSAI LAK-LEN SHAY-GYI ME-LONG (THE CRYSTAL MIRROR OF THE PRACTICE OF MOXABUSTION), self-published, undated. Xerox copies of this text were distributed by Norbu Rinpoche in Conway, MA at a moxabustion seminar in the fall of 1983. The text is handwritten in U-CHEN.

[6] Quote by Namkhai Norbu from an unspecified Tibetan astrological text, Conway, MA, Fall 1983

[7] Chu, W.K., trans. & Sherrill, W.A., ed., THE ASTROLOGY OF THE I CHING, Samuel Weiser, NY, 1980, p. 12

[8] COMMON TERMS OF TRADITIONAL CHINESE MEDICINE IN ENGLISH, by committee, Beijing Medical College, 1980, p. 425-426

[9] Ingredients in JIA WEI XIAO YAO TANG:

- Bupleurum
- Tang Kuei
- Peony
- Moutan
- Gardenia
- Atractylodes
- Poria
- Treated Licorice

OMENS OF DEATH

Reflections on Synchronicity in Medical Practice

Chinese medicine is based on the essential unity or holism of all existence and experience. This extends to the realm of Space/Time. The import of synchronicity is taken for granted in traditional Chinese culture. Synchronicity is the basis for such systems of prognostication as the I JING which is perhaps the single most important book in the history of Chinese culture. In the Tang and Song dynasties, due to the influence of Buddhism, much attention was paid by Chinese scholar-philosophers to the development of cosmology. Out of this same movement came Wang Ping's astrological chapters appended to his edition of the NEI JING, other systems of prognostication such as the several created by Shao Yung, and Dou Han-jing's ZU WU LIU CHU system of astrologically-timed "open" points. All these are based on the fundamental, mystical insight that any two phenomena arising at the same time are related since they were both caused by the same macrocosmic energies manifesting at that time. Therefore one can interpret the meaning of one, otherwise opaque phenomenon by infering a similar meaning as that of a more transparent simultaneous phenomenon.

In Chinese medicine, considerations involving time in diagnosis, treatment, and prognosis are an advanced level of practice. This is a level of practice that cannot be fully appreciated until one has had personal experience of the validity of mystical, as opposed to rational, experience. Therefore, critics operating from a purely rational mode of thought cannot adequately assess the truth of theories and techniques based on experiences of a higher level of reality they have not had. Such experiences are "scientifically" reproducible if one is willing to undego the training required. Such trainings are an integral part of the education of many lineages of traditional Oriental medicine. Generations of practitioners have experienced for themselves the validity of these higher levels of reality the same way that a person who has tasted sugar knows it is sweet. Such methods of training have been refined like well-honed experiments over no less than four millenia in Asia. However, just as one cannot expect to get the result from an experiment whose parameters have been altered to fit personal convienience, one cannot experience these higher dimensions of reality unless one undegoes such training as it has been pragmatically developed.

Contemporary Traditional Chinese Medicine, as taught in colleges in the People's Republic of China and at schools patterned after these in the West, in its attempt to mimic so-called scientific, i.e. materialist, procedure, has largely expunged this level of Chinese medical practice from its literature. Although there is a renewed interest in such theories and techniques as the ZU WU LIU CHU LIAO FA and the LING GUEI PA FA, the methodology adopted in state-sponsored clinics in China concerning the diagnosis and treatment of patients and the recording and writing of case histories leaves little, if any, room for such non-materialist considerations. In its attempt to look like western medicine, Chinese medicine runs the risk of cutting itself off from the springs of profundity which have made it great. Because of China's current economic and educational situation, many Chinese practitioners are not aware, as are a growing number of westerners, of the limitations and liabilities of so-called modern western medicine. Likewise, because of the purges of the Cultural Revolution, they have not had the opportunity to experience the pragmatic, clinically applicable wisdom of the old masters who had undegone the type of trainings described above. One has only to read the typical articles in the SHANGHAI JOURNAL OF ACUPUNCTURE & MOXABUSTION or the JOURNAL OF THE AMERICAN COLLEGE OF TRADITIONAL CHINESE MEDICINE to see how pervasive the influence of western methodology has been on the contemporary practice of TCM.

However, in my practice of Chinese medicine, I am continually reminded of the truth of synchronicity and for myself it seems apparent that my development as a healer to a great extent depends upon my ability to nurture this understanding. I have noticed all too often the effects of the phases of the moon, the weather, and the seasons on my patients to be content not to fudge these factors into their diagnoses and treatment. Likewise I have learned the hard way that everything a patient says and does in my presence is pregnant with meaning. Robert Tichy, a Denver acupuncturist, goes so far to say that patients literally tell him which points to use if he but listens carefully. I no longer discount any symptom the patient choses to share with me because it does not fit the diagnosis I have so far constructed. Each time I have, I have always been proven wrong. Too many times also, patients will report that they burned their herbs, misplaced them, broke their container, or that they spoiled at exactly the time that their symptoms underwent a change, in which case those herbs would have been inappropriate. Technically such revelatory occurences are called omens.[1]

As stated above, modern Chinese medical literature has little to say about omens. Tibetan medicine, on the other hand, has a great deal to say. The study of omenology is an integral part of the Tibetan physician's training. In the preeminent classic of Tibetan medicine, the GYUD ZHI, there is a section on omenology. This is in the DUD-TSI NYING-GYUD, the AMBROSIA HEART TANTRA[2]. These teachings are presented under the heading "Omens of Death". Since, from a single life-time's point of view, death is the worst prognosis, this section is basically about prognosis. Before, however, examining Tibetan lore on such omens, we must first briefly look at the Tibetan medical view on death itself.

According to Tibetan belief, there are two types of death: natural and accidental. At the moment of conception, caused on a spiritual level by karma from past lives, a maximum length of life is foreordained. This is analogous to the Chinese concept of the YUAN or Source Qi being finite at birth. When this energy is exhausted, death is inevitable and inescapable. No therapy, either medicinal or spiritual, can extend the life once this energy is used up. This is similar to the burning out of the wax of a candle and is what Tibetans refer to as natural death. Accidental death is due to any one of numerous adventitious causes snuffing out the candle flame even though there is plenty of wax left. Tibetan medicine describes such adventitious causes as imbalances in the Five Elements, the Three Humors, trauma, spiritual assault or possession, etc. In Chinese medicine these would be described likewise as various imbalances in the Elements, Organs, Humors, and Merdians and the effects of various sorts of trauma. Such adventitious imbalances or occurences can be forestalled or rectified with proper treatment, both remedial and preventive, as long as the basic life-force, what Tibetans call the SOG, still has fuel left to burn.

If a Tibetan doctor knows that a patient is near to death because of the omens, he can, if that death is adventitious, employ remedies to stave off that event. If that death is, on the other hand, due to an irreversible exhaustion of the patient's life-force, the doctor will instead concentrate on fascilitating a good death. This is based on the Tibetan doctor's almost always being a Spiritual Teacher or Lama. In such cases, the Lama-doctor's responsibility extends beyond death through the Intermediate State or BAR-DO to the patient's eventual rebirth. Tibetan Buddhist medicine includes, therefore, techniques for affecting the patient's experience in the BAR-DO and for helping secure a favorable rebirth.

Tibetan medicine also recognizes the importance of and places great store in the patient's belief in their doctor and the therapy he prescribes. Consequently, it consciously employs methods to build and consolidate this positive mental attitude. Therefore, the doctor's reputation is believed to be part of his or her ability as a healer. If one could know ahead of time whether or not they personally will be able to help a given patient, this would help preserve and bolster the doctor's reputation and therefore, it is believed by Tibetan doctors, their ability to heal. Successes create good word of mouth and failures detract from one's reputation. By studying the omens, a doctor can decide whether or not they have a positive karmic connection with a particular patient and whether that patient is likely to get better. Should the omens prove unfavorable, the doctor does not necessarily refuse treatment altogether but would refer the patient to another doctor with whom the patient may have a better karmic relationship.

This is not in any way a lack of compassion on the part of the doctor who is, in the Tibetan tradition, supposed to have taken the Bodhisattvic vow. Rather it is a sophisticated way of allocating resources so that everyone, especially the patient, benefits. There is no real purpose to be served if one knows that the case is hopeless or that, in any case, oneself is not the right doctor for a particular patient. The ability to make such a judgement at the beginning of a considered therapeutic relationship ultimately will save the patient time, money, and energy. Likewise it preserves the doctor's reputation which can be put to good use in more receptive patients and conserves the doctor's energy and equipoise, both of which are powers used in the healing encounter.

Therefore, according to the DUD-TSI NYING-GYUD, the first group of "omens of death" are called "distant". This means that the prognosis is unfavorable.

However it does not mean the patient necessarily is near death. I regard this type of omen as merely a sign that a particular doctor will not be able to help a particular patient. These omens are "read" either when the doctor is initally contacted or is on his way to the patient. In reading through the following lists, one must keep in mind that these omens relate to a particularly Tibetan and Buddhist cultural matrix and in our cultural milieu we should expect omens to fit our cultural prejudices and beliefs.

The omen is auspicious if the messenger sent to fetch the doctor is a Buddhist monk or other morally or spiritually exemplary person. The omen is unfavorable if the messenger is a woman, a cripple, comes riding on a buffalo, is trembling, frightened, panting, or holding a stone or fruitless branch, commits an evil act, sees or hears of a calamity on their way, is wearing ornaments of the opposite sex, is carrying weapons or other signs of death and destruction, or speaks rudely or disparagingly to the doctor or his servants.

The omen is also inauspicious if the messenger or call comes when the doctor is engaged in coarse thoughts or behavior, when cutting hair, wood, or anything else, when pulling down or dismantling a house, or when performing a fire puja. Likewise, it is inauspicious if the messenger started out for the doctor or the patient calls on the sixth, fourth, or nineth days of the lunar month. The sixteenth, twenty-sixth, fouteenth, twenty-fourth, nineteenth, and twentieth are also inauspicious to a lesser extent. Solar and lunar eclipses are also deemed inauspicious, as are bad stellar influences and generally at night.

If the doctor must travel to the patient, it is an inauspicious omen of unfavorable prognosis if he encounters cutting or breaking of anything, hears or sees weeping or killing or any other calamities, if a cat, monkey, otter, or snake crosses his path, or if he sees a cripple, an accident, or any evil deed. However, the prognosis is favorable if, on the other hand, he encounters a meritorious act, a religious ritual, full vessels of grain or yogurt, lamps, flowers, or offerings, gold, jewels, a person engaged in spiritual practice, images of divine beings, horses, sheep, or cattle with young, or fried rice or jam. And finally, if the doctor sees a fire die without a wind or yogurt or alcohol are brought out of the house of the patient just as the doctor arrives, the prognosis is unfavorable.

If one thinks about these omens, the favorable ones all have to do with wealth, health, growth, fecundity, and abundance. Whereas the unfavorable ones all have to do with decay, death, decline, and debility. Nor is such a list meant to be exhaustive. Rather the practitioner should regard such a list as merely examples of commonly accepted inauspicious omens in that culture. What is important is that the doctor should be mindful of anything he or she sees, hears, or thinks when the patient calls up for an appointment or experiences on the way to the patient's bedside. Since the beginnings of things presage how they will grow and develop, attention should be paid to the intial contact between patient and practitioner as in the first appointment. However, inauspicious omens may arise at any point in the relationship counselling the termination of that relation.

In my own experience, a positive omen has been the sun coming out from behind the clouds when talking to a prospective patient. A negative omen has been my son's dropping a glass of milk on the floor while talking to another. Also I have found from experience that I cannot successfully treat any woman with a particular name. This is based on numerous misadventures with bearers of this name in the past and also on several historical incidents with my Teachers with women of this name. Therefore I now refer all patients with this name to another practitioner.

This may sound superstitious to those of a materialist frame of mind. However, I have found such omens in my own practice to be highly revelatory. When I pay attention to such omens, I and the patient benefit. When I disregard such intimations, I have always suffered the consequences, either sooner or later. Happily, it is only the exceptional cases where omens, in fact, present themselves. Most cases are not, I find, attended by omens. Omens are merely a sign that more care must be taken. It is these "distant omens of death" which I think are most important on a day to day basis and to which the traditional Oriental physician needs to pay attention.

The second class of distant omens are dreams. Depending upon the contents of the patient's dreams, the prognosis is more or less favorable. In the Tibetan literature, the list of inauspicious dream subjects and scenarios are again a reflection of specifically Tibetan Buddhist cultural values. The following list is not meant to be definitive. Western practitioners need to examine their patients' dreams in the light of both their and their patients' cultural expectations and belief systems. Since we live in a heterodox society, this is no easy matter.

The following dreams are all considered inauspicious by Tibetan standards: riding a cat, monkey, tiger, fox, or corpse; riding a buffalo naked to the south; a willow tree with a bird's nest growing out of the top of one's head; a thorny tree growing out of one's Heart; lotuses emerging from one's Heart; falling from a cliff; sleeping in a cemetery; one's head breaking open; being surrounded by crows and carrion eaters; dreaming of beasts which eat their young such as scorpions; skin peeling off one's limbs; entering one's mother's womb; being carried away by a river; being stuck in a swamp; being swallowed by a fish; losing in trade or a quarrel; wishing to dance; taking a bride; having one's hair and beard shaved; drinking with deceased friends and relatives; wearing red clothes and garlands; and dancing with deceased acquaintances. If a sick person continually has such dreams it forebodes a bad prognosis. If an otherwise healthy person habitually has such dreams, it means that some impediment to their life has arisen which may be circumvented by the proper <u>spiritual</u> remedies.

Not all dreams are necessarily premonitory. In general, Tibetans believe that dreams which are forgotten produce no result. It is only dreams which are very clearly experienced and which are remembered upon arising that may have a premonitory meaning. Dreams recapitualing some event from the preceding day, or replaying what one has seen or heard, dreams arising from some ailment, such as dreaming of being burnt during a high fever, such dreams all have no premonitory power or import.

Auspicious dreams which augur a favorable prognosis are: of a diety; of holy or famous personages; of a huge buffalo; of a flame burning unobstructedly; a lake overflowing; blood or filth smeared on the <u>outside</u> of one's body; wearing white clothes; raising a "banner of victory" or a "royal umbrella"; receiving fruit; climbing a mountain; dreaming of a fine horse or a tree laden with fruit; riding an elephant, lion, horse, or cow; crossing a river or an ocean; escaping from misery or prison; travelling towards the northeast; and being praised by a diety or one's parents. If an otherwise sick person has such auspicious dreams, it is a sign that he or she will recover even though their symptoms may still be severe. This corresponds to the Chinese medical belief that a patient whose SHEN is intact is likely to recover even though suffering from an otherwise dangerous disease.

The last type of distant omen is when one "for no apparent reason" hates their doctor, nurse, friends, relatives, medicine, and/or their spiritual guide. This is an inauspicious omen. It is more serious in an ill person than in a healthy one. It is obvious that little help can be expected from a treatment, doctor, or guide one has no faith in or detests. I have personally found that I do not obtain favorable results in patients with whom I do not have a friendly and pleasant rapport. If I feel even from our first phone conversation that I will not be able to "get along" with a prospective patient nor they with me, I know now to refer them to another practitioner. Some personalities do not mesh. However, for a good therapeutic result to be obtained I have found a positive rapport is almost always necessary.

In the DUD-TSI NYING-GYUD, there is a final group of miscellaneous distant omens. These include fading complexion, constant depression, crows refusing to eat one's left-over offerings, water not remaining on one's chest after a bath, no sound being produced when the fingernails are clicked together, becoming weaker no matter what one eats, changes in one's body odor, change in the number of body lice, dulling of sexual desire, changes in temper, and no shadow appearing in the water or a mirror. Some of these omens are peculiar and I have no explanation or rationalization for them. Others can be accounted for reasonably. Changes in the body odor and lice imply a weakening of host energy allowing for increased growth of parasites. Becoming weaker no matter what or how much one eats suggests diabetes. Dulling of the sexual desire indicates Kidney Yang Deficiency. Changes in temper, implying the patient's becoming more impatient, suggest Liver Yang elevation, Heart Fire, or Yin Deficiency, i.e. Internal patterns of disharmony potentially leading to death.

The next major group of omens listed in the DUD-TSI NYING-GYUD are called "near" omens. These are further divided into near and extremely near categories. Under near omens are listed hemorrhaging from any of the body's orifices, immediately forgetting what has been said, and retraction of the penis and scrotum. Hemorrhaging indicates the Spleen's inability to hold the Blood, upsurging of Yang, and/or Hot Blood. Forgetting immediately what has just been said indicates Kidney JING Deficiency and/or Spleen Deficiency.

If an otherwise healthy person experiences any of the following near omens, it means there is an impediment to their life-force which may result in death in sixth months or so. These include making a strange noise when clearing the throat or sneezing, not smelling the odor of a lamp going out, no sensation when one's hair is pulled out, the appearance of an oily exudate on the crown of one's head, new parts or swirls in the hair or eyebrows, lines like "new moons" around the eyes or lips, perceiving more or less with any of the senses, not being able to see one's own wrist when touching the top of their head, lack of luster of the eye whites "like a sleeping rabbit", loss of color in the pupils, ears sticking to the sides of the head, absence of a roar inside the ears when cupped with the hands, and "no shadow from vapor arising from the head".

These last mentioned omens are themselves quite opaque and need an oral commentary on them by an experienced Tibetan doctor to ellucidate them. All I can say is that several years ago one of my Teachers told me that I might die that year and that a serious impediment to my life had arisen due to the ripening of past bad karma. Several months later, the swirl in my hair at the back of my head changed sides. Several months after that I almost did die. However, other near omens of death are more easily understood from the point of view of Chinese medicine. These include flaring of the nostrils, darkening of the center strip of the tongue, drying and shortening of the tongue, the lower lip drooping down while the upper lip curls up, the facial complexion becoming blotchy, the breath becoming cold and the teeth dark, the disappearance of bodily heat, and the breath coming in gasps. These last two omens indicate the dying of the Fire of Life, the MING MEN HUO, and the Kidneys' inability to grasp the Qi in the QI HAI. Drying and shortening of the tongue indicates the Qi and Blood of the Five ZHANG are extremely depleted.

The extremely near omens correspond to the stages of the actual process of dying. The eye organ diminishes and loses its ability to see. The ear organ diminshes and loses its ability to hear. Then the nose loses the ability to smell, the tongue loses taste, the tactile sense loses touch, and the mind loses consciousness. As the Earth element sinks into Water, vision is lost. As the Water sinks into Fire, the orifices become dry. When Fire sinks into Wind or Air, bodily heat is lost. When Wind sinks into Space, breathing stops. After death, depending upon any discharge from the body orifices, one can determine in which of the Six Realms of Samsara the patient's karma will cause them to be reborn.

Lastly there are two other categories of omens of death. These are "uncertain" omens and "certain" ones. Uncertain omens accompany disease. These can include either distant or near omens. If the disease is cured and the omens desist, there is no further impediment to the patient's life. If, however, the disease is "cured" but the omens persist, the prognosis is poor since the impediment to life has not, in fact, been eliminated. This corresponds to a disease undergoing transformation or becoming latent. The novice physician might assume the disease has been cured when it really hasn't. According to the NEI JING, diseases undergo transformations due to seasonal influences and can cause death one or two seasons later. Certain omens refer to the clear diagnostic signs that the bodily constituents are disordered to the point of coming apart. In Chinese terms this relates to the irreparable separation of Yin and Yang.

According to the DUD-TSI NYING-GYUD, "one may reverse the omens of death with regard to dreams, character, distant, and uncertain omens by collecting religious merit, etc. For near and certain omens, save the lives of animals that are destined to be killed. There are no methods for reversing extremely close omens."[3] This advice for reversing the omens of death means that on top of correct medical diagnosis and treatment one should also ameliorate their situation by consciously creating fresh good karma to bolster their life-force. This, in turn, is based on the Tibetan medical concept that there are two levels of the causation of disease. The first is called the ultimate level. On this level, disease, a species of suffering, in fact one of the four great rivers of suffering of the human realm,[4] is the result of the ripening of effects of unvirtuous behavior or bad karma. It is said in Tibetan that bad karma has only one good quality which is that, until it comes to fruition, it can be altered or eradicated by the antidote of virtuous behavior or good karma. The second level of disease is called the proximate level. This is the level of the interrelationship between the Organs, Humors, Elements, and the macrocosmic energies and cycles. The proximate cause of disease is the phenomenal manifestation of the ultimate cause. On the proximate level, disease is treated by herbs, acupuncture, surgery, massage, etc. However, these can only be effective if there is the good karma to support a recovery. The omens of death are one way of ascertaining if the karmic cause for recovery exists. If not, within certain limitations, this karmic deficiency can be made up.

When several years ago, my Teacher prognosticated that I might die that year and then almost did due to a Heart imbalance, she told me that although my length of life should be reasonably long, my present difficulties were due to bad karma created as a youth ripening at this point in my life. As a youngster and teenager I was very fond of killing all manner of animals and bugs and of hunting and fishing. I went to a number of doctors, none of whom were able to treat me. I tried treating myself but to no avail. Although I learned a great deal of Chinese medicine in my researching my symptoms and syndrome, nothing I did made much difference in my ill health. My Teacher prescribed certain religious practices for the purification of bad karma and the creation of good karma pertaining to the life-force. It was only these that made any significant improvement in my condition. Two years later, another Lama doctor took my pulse and was able to read this whole occurence. He likewise prescribed similar religous practices for the accumulation of life-merit without his previously knowing anything about my history. At the same time that my Teacher prognosed that I was out of immanent danger, I had several dreams exactly corrsponding to several of the auspicious dreams listed above reversing the previous ill omens.

Contemporary TCM speaks only of the proximate cause and treatment of disease. However classical Chinese medicine has always included lineages with a more holistic theory incorporating the spiritual as well as the mundane. Such lineages are most commonly found amongst Buddhist and Taoist practitioners. However, even the Neo-confuscianists who were responsible for the great theoretical advances in Chinese medicine of the Song, Jin, Yuan, and Ming dynasties were essentially mystics. That the ultimate causes of health and disease were recognized by some classical Chinese doctors is evidenced by the following statements by Ge Hung: "Accordingly, when we examine the moral injunctions of the various teachings, we find all of them agreeing that those desiring Fullness of Life must strive to accumulate goodness, win merit, be kind and affectionate to others, practice the Golden Rule, love even the creeping things, rejoice in the good fortune of others and commiserate with their sufferings, help those in distress and the poor, harm no living thing, utter no curse, look upon the successes and failures of others as their own, not be proud, not vaunt themselves, not envy their betters, and conceal no evil intentions with flattery. In this way they become men of exalted character and receive good fortune from heaven. Their undertakings are[5] sure to be successful, and they can seek ("immortality") with hope of success."

In the BAR-DO THO-DROL, the so-called TIBETAN BOOK OF THE DEAD, additional omens are listed. These are divided into outer, inner, secret, and distant categories. However, many of these omens are the products of consciously practiced yogic procedures. These practices cannot be learned from a book nor should they be attempted without proper oral transmission, initiation, and explanation from an authorized Teacher holding their living lineage. Without fulfilling these requirements, one will not be able to make these practices work. In general, these practices are not taught to novices. I practiced for fifteen years under my Teachers before any of them were ever taught to me.

Traditional Chinese Medicine has diagnostic signs analogous to the Tibetan certain omens. There are the Seven Death pulses and the Seven Critical tongues. The Seven Death pulses are like 1) shrimps swimming, 2) birds pecking, 3) recoiling from a stone, 4) a fish swaying, 5) a boiling pot, 6) rain dripping from the edge of a roof, and 7) a loose rope. The Seven Critical tongues indicate 1) Yin Qi dying, 2) Fluids dried up, 3) Fluids absent, 4) Collapse of Blood circulation, 5) Liver Qi dying, 6) Renal Qi dying, and 7) Yang Qi dying. Their descriptions can be found in "Tongue Diagnosis" by Yang Chih-yi.[6] Near death can also be prognosed by the absence of a post-tibial pulse in a seriously ill patient or a hard mass at QI HAI (CV 6) in a patient in extremis. Both are signs of immanent exit. However, it is not such signs of near death, whether Chinese or Tibetan, which are potentially the most thought-provoking.

It is my belief that the distant omens concerning the intial contact betwen patient and practitioner are the most pregnant for practitioners of contemporary TCM. By allowing the possible validity of such omens, practitioners may also become encouraged to investigate other aspects of "spiritual" medicine currently excluded from modern TCM practice but very much a part of such a highly developed and clinically effective system as Tibetan medicine. These would include all aspects of temporality and synchronicity vis a vis diagnosis, treatment and prognosis. This might also include attention to the ultimate or ethical causes of disease, demonic interference or possession, TIAN BING or Heavenly retribution disease, the psychospiritual empowerment of medications, the use of ritual in treatment, and the development of healing power within the practitioner beyond theoretical concepts and techniques.

Contemporary TCM's attempted mimickry of so-called scientific medicine's methodology is to me a bad omen. Western scientific or allopathic medicine's rejection by a growing segment of the population is due to its materialist tunnel vision. In its attempt to reduce the multi-dimensional fabric of reality to a mechanistic, materialistic thread, it cuts itself off from the source of life. It is my hope that American practitioners, seeing the limitations and plight of allopathy, may stem this trend in contemporary Chinese medicine. This does not mean jettisoning the rigor and rationality of TCM diagnosis, the differentiation of syndromes, the deducing of treatment principles, or the logical erection of treatment plans. It means adding to this rational level a suprarational or spiritual perspective, which, once accepted or experienced, is totally logical and consistent within itself, to ensure our system's connection with Heaven.

ENDNOTES

1 The Tibetan word for omen is TEN-DREL. This is a Buudhist philosophical meaning coemergent. The TEN-DREL CHU-NYIS are the twelve links of causal coemergence known in Sanskrit as the PRATITYASAMUTPADA. The Tibetan word clearly implies interdependence, coproduction, and simultaneous arising from a complex but unified matrix. Whenever a happy coincidence is perceived, it is common for Tibetans to say, "TEN-DREL YAK-PO DUK" which means the coemergence is auspicious. In English, however, we would more likely say is it a good omen.

2 THE AMBROSIA HEART TANTRA (DUD-TSI NYING-GYUD), Yeshi Donden, annotator; Jhampa Kelsang, trans., Library of Tibetan Works & Archives, Dharamsala, India, 1977

3 Ibid. p. 75

4 According to Buddhism, in fact, according to Lord Buddha Himself, there are ten ways of creating bad karma as a human being. These are divided into three groups. The first group of three refer to unvirtuous behavior performed by the body. They are killing or physically harming any sentient being, taking what has not been freely given, and sexual misconduct, which includes adultery, rape, incest, or any other sexual act committed without free consent or causing harm or pain to another. The second group of four refer to unvirtuous utterances of speech. These are lying, slander, abusive language, and gossip, all of which may cause harm to another. The third group of three refer to unvirtuous thoughts. They include ill will towards another sentient being, such as wishing them dead or injured, coveting another's possessions, or having views about the nature of reality and therefore about the Teacher, Buddha, Dharma, Sangha contrary to the Dharma. An example of such a wrong view is the opinion that there is no such thing as karma and therefore that one can do anything without inescapable reaction.

Buddhists believe that committing any of the above ten unvirtuous actions lead to rebirth in one of the three lower realms, i.e. as a denizen of hell, a hungry ghost, or an animal depending upon the severity of the commission and the motivation. If the act is not severe enough to lead to such a rebirth or if its consequences have been largely experienced already and only a lesser residuum remains, the person may experience a reaction, either in this life or a future one as a human being. In this case, the reaction will be logically related to the nature of the transgression or harm experienced by another. Therefore, the karmic reaction to killing is to have one's own life cut short or endangered.

5 Ge Hung, ALCHEMY, MEDICINE, RELIGION IN THE CHINA OF A.D. 320 (PAO PU TZU NIE PIEN), James R. Ware, trans., MIT Press, Cambridge & London, 1966, p. 116

6 Yang Chih-yi, "Tongue Diagnosis", BULLETIN OHAI, LA, Vol. 6, # 1, 1981, p. 42

ON BEING AT THE RIGHT PLACE AT THE WRONG TIME

An Investigation into the Astrological Proscriptions of Classical Acupuncture

> The eastern neighbor who slaughters an ox is not as much in harmony with the time as the western neighbor. The latter attains true happiness (and) good fortune comes in great measure.[1]

Thus reads the judgement for nine in the fifth place of Hexagram 63, After Completion, of the I JING. As Helmut Willhelm explains, "The difference in the outcome of the sacrifice depends not on the attitude of the sacrificer as one might expect but on the timing of the sacrifice."[2]

In recent years there has been a resurgence of interest in traditional Chinese medical astrology in relation to picking so-called Open points. Although this interest is encouraging, since it implies a renewed interest in the deeper and more esoteric levels of Chinese medicine, appreciation for and research into the Closed points, in my opinion, hold even deeper insights. Many contemporary practitioners of Chinese medicine have become fixated on the alleviation of symptoms as their main concern. Classical Chinese medical writings have typically held, however, that symptomatic treatment is not as important as preventive treatment. Because our modern lifestyle is based on immediate gratification we often seek only quick fixes for our problems and ignore such solutions' long-term implications. Too often modern practitioners groping for more effective immediate treatments grasp at the simple certainty of an Open point. Such an approach is especially attractive in cases where the diagnosis is complex. On the one hand, employment of an astrological Open point may tap a deeper level of macro-microcosmic imbalance. But on the the other, it might also be used as an excuse for a lack of deep understanding of classical medical theory and an accurate diagnosis from which an exact and logical treatment can be deduced. Understanding the rationale and implications of Closed points, however, immediately forces us to consider the long-range and subtle effects of our treatments.

Although the calculations for determining both auspicious and inauspicious moments for acupuncture first proliferated during the late Tang and Song dynasties under the influence of both Buddhism and Neoconfucianism, it was not until the thirteenth century that Dou Han-jing authored the two works that are considered the loci classici of this science of timing acupuncture based on astrology. They were the ZI WU LIU CHU (THE NOON & MIDNIGHT DIFFERENCES IN THE FLOW OF QI) and the DOU TAI SHU XIAN SUNG LIU CHU FU (MASTER DOCTOR DOU ON THE CIRCULATION OF QI). Written between 1230 and 1240, these texts outlined not only the hourly rhythms of Qi flow but also daily, monthly, and seasonal circuits.

By the Ming dynasty, astrological considerations were a generally accepted part of clinical practice. A preface written by Jin Li-meng in a work of that period, the ZHEN JIU ZI RI PIEN, is quite clear on this point: "Therefore the classical manuals of acupuncture say that if you know the right time to apply it, an illness is bound to be cured. But, if you miss the hour, diseases are difficult to deal with. So there is nothing more important in acupuncture and moxabustion than to choose the right moment."[3] Although Jin Li-meng's statement exemplifies both the classical and contemporary emphasis on determining the right place and time to administer treatment, implicit in this notion is that there are as well wrong times and places for treatment. Since our first injunction as healers is to first do no harm, attention to proscribed times and places should logically be equally as important.

The ZHEN JIU DA CHENG (THE GREAT COMPENDIUM OF ACUPUNCTURE & MOXABUSTION) published in 1601 by Yang Ji-zhou contains a fairly complex section on just such proscriptions. As a compiler, Yang Ji-zhou drew his material from a number of sources all held in high regard at that point in time. At the time of its publication, such astrological considerations had already passed the peak of their vogue and were beginning to come under criticism as being clinically unverifiable and unwieldy. Yang was an adherent of the LING YI school, the school of clinical practice as opposed to the JU YI or Confucian Scholastic school. While LING YI practitioners often had a reputation for rather careless scholarship, their writings were always grounded in solid clinical experience. Happily for us, Yang's genius seems to have bridged both schools. Although the clinical applicability of the material presented in the ZHEN JIU DA CHENG is stressed, it is presented in a clear and organized manner reflecting a scholarly concern as well. Given Yang Ji-zhou's background as primarily a clinician and the nature of the DA CHENG itself (considered by many to be one of the most important works on acupuncture in the medical canon) as a compendium of practically essential acupuncture knowledge, it would seem odd that Yang would include a section on astrological acupuncture if it were based on numerical superstition and was without clinical value. The presence of this material in the ZHEN JIU DA CHENG is for me an endorsement of its potential clinical value.

Below are the major astrological proscriptions against acupuncture taken from the ZHEN JIU DA CHENG. These have been supplemented by several other proscriptions taken from other sources for completeness' sake. Sources other than the DA CHENG are indicated in the text. But before we can make sense immediately of these lists of proscribed times, we must first understand something about Chinese astrology itself.

Chinese "astrology" is not like its western counterpart. In fact, it is not so much concerned with the movements of the planets and other heavenly bodies as it is with a numerological system of smaller cycles of time within larger cycles of time. The basis for this numerology is the Sexagenary cycle produced by combining the Ten Celestial Stems (TIAN GAN) with the Twelve Terrestial Branches (DI ZHI). This Sexagenary cycle is the most ancient Chinese method of counting the days, extending back to the second millenium BCE. This same Sexagenary cycle has been used to count the years since the first century BCE. In fact, it predates both the lunar and solar calendrical systems in China.[4] There is, in addition, a ten day circuit corresponding to the Ten Celestial Stems, while the Twelve Terrestial Branches are used to count the months of the year and the hours of the day. Below we have used the following notation for identifying the Stems and Branches: S refers to the Stem, while B refers to the Branch. S-5 means the fifth Stem out of ten and B-11 means the eleventh Branch out of twelve. Therefore, when Stem and Branch are combined, as they commonly are to make up the Sexagenary cycle, they will appear as S-5 B-11 or WU XU, the thirty-fifth segment of the Sexagenary cycle. For a more complete exposition on the use of Stems and Branches in Chinese medicine, the reader is recommended to see Manfred Porkert's THE THEORETICAL FOUNDATIONS OF CHINESE MEDICINE.[5]

Proscriptions forbidding acupuncture on certain regions of the body occur based on yearly, seasonal, monthly, daily, and hourly cycles. Some of these cycles overlap and combine two separate cycles. Beginning with the yearly cycle, there is a list of proscriptions in the DA CHENG called the JIU GONG KAO SHEN JIN JI or the Nine House KAO SHEN contraindications. These proscriptions are based on the Eight Trigrams. Each of the Eight Trigrams and a "middle house" relating to the number five correspond to one year within a nine year cycle. This is based on the so-called Magic Square. Each Trigram in turn corresponds to a body part or parts which are thus "forbidden" to needle during each respective year. As the DA CHENG says: "In the first year KUN arises and in the second year CHEN and so on through the years throughout the circuit and finally returning to the beginning. Moving through the years and in all places it is this circuit which governs bodily injury and the prohibitions for acupuncture and moxabustion. If one inadvertently disregards this and <u>even lightly</u> treats prohibited areas, ulcers will develop. While if these areas are treated strongly, then death ensues. Guard against this!"[6] The entire nine year cycle is as follows:

KUN	Heel
CHEN	Gastrocnemius, Fingers, and Teeth
SUN	Head, Breast, and Mouth
ZHONG GONG (middle house)	Shoulder and Buttocks
QIAN	Back and Eyes
DUI	Arms and Hands
GEN	Neck and Lumbar region
LI	Knees and Ribs
KAN	Elbows, Legs, and Abdomen

Moxabustion is also proscribed at certain areas of the body likewise based on a yearly cycle. However, according to the HUANG TI MING TANG JIU JING (THE YELLOW EMPEROR'S MOXA CLASSIC), these prohibitions are based on the Twelve Terrestial Branches plus the age of the patient. The YELLOW EMPEROR'S MOXA CLASSIC states that certain areas or organs are "unsuitable" for

for moxabustion treatment during certain years and ages due to the location of the SHEN there at those times.[7] In applying this system of prohibitions it should be remembered that according to traditional oriental methods of reckoning one's age, one is one year old at birth and everyone advances one year in age on the seventh day of the first lunar month no matter what solar day they actually were born on.

SHEN resides in:	Moxa is prohibited at these areas in these ages:							
Heart	1	13	25	37	49	61	73	85
Throat	2	14	26	38	50	62	74	86
Head	3	15	27	39	51	63	75	87
Eyebrows	4	16	28	40	52	64	76	88
Back	5	17	29	41	53	65	77	89
Lumbar region	6	18	30	42	54	66	78	90
Abdomen	7	19	31	43	55	67	79	91
Back of the neck	8	20	32	44	56	68	80	92
Legs	9	21	33	45	57	69	81	93
Knees	10	22	34	46	58	70	82	94
YIN (the genitalia)	11	23	35	47	59	71	83	95
Thigh	12	24	36	48	60	72	84	96

While not arranged in the DA CHENG in this order, let us next consider seasonal proscriptions since these are next in line in terms of a continuum of increasingly smaller and therefore more specific cycles. Yang Ji-zhou cites a series of cautions known as TAI YI which are also found in Chapter 78 of the LING SHU. These are not, strictly speaking, forbidden or contraindicated. However, a strong cautionary warning is given when treating with needles during these respective times. These precautions are as follows:

On the first day of Spring and on WU YIN S-5 B-3 days and JI CHOU S-6 B-2 days we caution in treating the left foot.

On the vernal equinox and on YI MAO S-2 B-4 days we caution in treating the left side of the chest and ribs.

On the first day of Summer and on WU CHEN S-5 B-5 days and JI SI S-6 B-6 days we caution treating the left hand.

On the summer solstice and BING WU S-3 B-7 days we should use caution in treating the chest, throat, head, and neck.

On the first day of Autumn and WU SHEN S-5 B-9 days as well as JI WEI S-6 B-8 days we use caution in treating the right hand.

On the autumnal equinox and on XIN YU S-8 B-10 days use caution in treating the right side of the chest and ribs.

On the first day of Winter and WU XI S-5 B-11 days and JI HAI S-6 B-12 days use caution in treating the right foot.

During the winter solstice and REN ZI S-9 B-1 days we use caution in treating the sexual organs, lumbar region, and buttocks.

These cautions are further summarized in a section known as SI JI REN SHEN (The Personal Spirit of the Four Seasons): "In the Spring and Autumn one finds the place of the Spirit in the left and right sides. In Winter and Summer one finds the place of the Spirit in the lumbar region and the umbilicus. Use extreme caution with acupuncture and moxabustion (in these places at these times)."[8]

There are then specific days during which acupuncture should be avoided according to the season. This enumeration is called SI JI BI JI RI or Days to Avoid Acupuncture According to the Season.[9] As listed in the DA CHENG they are:

During the Spring on JIA and YI, S-1 and S-2 days

During the Summer on BING and DING, S-3 and S-4 days

During the Autumn on GENG and XIN, S-7 and S-8 days

During the Winter on REN and GUI, S-9 and S-10 days

All the time on WU and JI, S-5 and S-6 days

Then , throughout the month there are periods determined by the waxing and maning of the moon during which certain therapeutic actions should not be undertaken. The ZHEN JIU DA CHENG in turns quotes Chapter 26 of the SU WEN for these proscriptions: "In practicing acupuncture one must attune oneself to the Qi of the Sun, Moon, and Stars, the Four Seasons, and the Eight ZHENG such that only when their Qi is settled may one needle. Thus, when it is warm and the sun is bright, one's Blood flows gently and with fluidity. When it is cold and the Sun is overcast, one's Blood congeals and the Qi sinks. As the Moon waxes, the Blood and Qi quicken and the WEI QI begins to move. While the Moon is full, the Blood and Qi are in flourescence and the flesh and sinews thrive. As the Moon wanes the tonus of the flesh and the sinews also diminishes, the channels and collaterals become Deficient, the WEI QI departs, and the body's form becomes hollow. Consequently, one must observe the seasonal changes in order to regulate the Qi and Blood. When the weather turns cold, do not needle. However, when the weather is warm, one needs not hestitate. When the Moon is waxing, do not drain. When the Moon is full do not tonify. And when the Moon is waning, one should not treat (with acupuncture) at all. This is known as treating in accordance with the seasons.

"Thus, when the Moon is waxing and one drains, the organs become Deficient, while when the Moon is full and one tonifies, the Qi and Blood are said to be replete, Blood stagnates in the LUO, and this is called a dual Excess. When the Moon is waning and one treats, this is said to disrupt the channels and the Yin and Yang become confused."[10]

Next, daily proscriptions are based on ten and twelve day cycles, the Sexagenary daily cycle, and the thirty day lunar cycle. First is a daily proscription according to the lunar cycle called ZHU RI REN SHEN or Daily Movements of the Personal

Spirit. Although this system of calculation appears in the much earlier HUANG TI MING TANG JIU JING, here it is specifically and unequivocally stated that the Personal Spirit resides in a particular body location on a particular day. The list of correspondences is as follows:[11]

Day 1 - Big toe	15 - One half of the body
2 - Lateral malleolus	16 - Stomach
3 - Inguinal joint	17 - QI CHONG (St 30)
4 - Lumbar region	18 - Thighs
5 - Mouth & tongue	19 - Feet
6 - Hands	20 - Medial malleolus
7 - Medial malleolus	21 - Little fingers
8 - Feet & arms	22 - Lateral malleolus
9 - Buttocks	23 - Liver & feet
10 - Back	24 - Hand Yang Ming
11 - Nose	25 - Foot Yang Ming
12 - Between front hairline & face	26 - Chest
13 - Teeth	27 - Knees
14 - Stomach	28 - "YIN"
29 - Knees	30 - Heels

The ten day cyclic prohibitions based on the Ten Celestial Stems are as follows:[12]

S-1	JIA	Head	S-6	JI	Spleen
S-2	YI	Throat	S-7	GENG	Lumbar region
S-3	BING	Shoulders	S-8	XIN	Knees
S-4	DING	Heart	S-9	REN	Kidneys
S-5	WU	Abdomen	S-10	GUI	Feet

The twelve days cyclic prohibitions based on the Twelves Terrestial Branches are:[13]

B-1	ZI	Eyes	B-7	WU	Heart
B-2	CHOU	Ears	B-8	WEI	Feet
B-3	YIN	Chest	B-9	SHEN	Head
B-4	MAO	Teeth	B-10	YU	Knees
B-5	CHEN	Lumbar region	B-11	XU	Lower YIN
B-6	SI	Hands	B-12	HAI	Neck

There is also another daily cycle based on the Sexagenary cycle combining the day and the patient's gender as well:[14]

NAN BI JI RI (DAYS TO AVOID TREATING MEN)

REN CHEN	S-9 B-5	PING WU	S-3 B-7
JAI CHEN	S-1 B-5	DING WEI	S-4 B-8
YI SI	S-2 B-6	XIN WEI	S-8 B-8

Also all XU days B-11

NU BI JI RI (DAYS TO AVOID TREATING WOMEN)

JAI YIN	S-1 B-3	YI SI	S-2 B-6
YI MAO	S-2 B-4	DING SI	S-4 B-6
YI YU	S-2 B-10	XIN WEI	S-8 B-8

And also all "unlucky days" and HAI days B-12

Chapter 61 of the HUANG TI NEI JING LING SHU warns against needling specific areas of the body on specific days according to the ten day cycle coordinated with the Celestial Stems. According to the author of the LING SHU, these are as follows:

On JIA S-1 and YI S-2 days caution in needling the head

On BING S-3 and DING S-4 days caution in needling the shoulder and throat

On WU S-5 and JI S-6 days caution in needling the abdomen

On GENG S-7 and XIN S-8 days caution in needling the thighs and knees

On REN S-8 and GUI S-10 days caution in needling the shins

Hourly proscriptions simply based on the Twelve Terrestial Branches are listed in the DA CHENG under the heading ZHU SHI REN SHEN or Hourly Movements of the Personal Spirit. [15]

ZI hour	11 PM - 1 AM	Ankle	WU hour	11 AM - 1 PM	Chest
CHOU hour	1 AM - 3 AM	Lumbar	WEI hour	1 PM - 3 PM	Abdomen
YIN hour	3 AM - 5 AM	Eyes	SHEN hour	3 PM - 5 PM	Heart
MAO hour	5 AM - 7 AM	Face	YU hour	5 PM - 7 PM	Back
CHEN hour	7 AM - 9 AM	Head	XU hour	7 PM - 9 PM	Neck
SU hour	9 AM - 11 AM	Hand	HAI hour	9 PM - 11 PM	Thighs

Interestingly the HUANG TI MING TANG JIU JING gives a very similar circuit specifically regarding moxabustion prohibitions.[16]

ZI hour	11 PM - 1 AM	Ankle	WU hour	11 AM - 1 PM	Chest
CHOU hour	1 AM - 3 AM	Head	WEI hour	1 PM - 3 PM	Abdomen
YIN hour	3 AM - 5 AM	Ears	SHEN hour	3 PM - 5 PM	Heart
MAO hour	5 AM - 7 AM	Face	YU hour	5 PM - 7 PM	Back
CHEN hour	7 AM - 9 AM	Neck	XU hour	7 PM - 9 PM	Lumbar
SU hour	9 AM - 11 AM	Breast	HAI hour	9 PM - 11 PM	Thighs

While the professional astrologer reading these lists of prohibitions and cautions may admire the complexity and seeming exactitude of all these classical Chinese computations, the modern clinical acupuncturist may very well throw up their hands in exasperation and lament that, if one were to take into account all of these overlapping proscriptions, no point of the body might ever be open. Certainly utilizing these various proscriptions makes the routine use of certain acupuncture formulae administered bilaterally every day or every other day, as is the contemporary trend in China, impossible.

On the one hand, this may be the very value of these lists of proscriptions. They demand an approach to acupuncture that is an immediate assessment of the Qi flowing in the various channels and collaterals at the distinct moment of treatment. In our modern world we assume that time is homogenous. However, in eastern thought and cosmology, moments in time are not homogenous or identical. An example of the variability of time in eastern thought is the Buddhist cosmological concept that the karmic or causal reaction of a similar action may be stronger or weaker at different moments of time. For instance, according to Buddhism, an action done during the first fifteen days of the first lunar month will result in a hundred thousandfold greater reaction than the same act committed on some other day. Days of special karmic potency or reactivity include the eighth, tenth, fifteenth, twenty-fifth, and thirtieth days of the lunar month which correspond to the phases of the Moon and the state of our internal energies. In terms of acupuncture this implies that the effect or result of needling a certain set of points on one day may not be the same as on another day. This likewise is the implication from the passage from the I JING quoted at the beginning of this essay. Such an appreciation of the qualitative and quantitative texture of time is foreign to our modern view colored by materialism. But, since the flow of Qi is responsive to and identical with the flow of Change on the ontological level, it is logical that acupuncture which proports to be the manipulation of this flow of Qi within the human body should pay close attention to the vagaries of time.

On the other hand, amongst this welter of prohibitions and cautions not all of these are of equal importance. Depending upon the diagnosis and the intentions of treatment and the mechanics of the treatment itself as it impinges upon the organism, some of these cyclic proscriptions are more important than others. According to the DA CHENG, the KAO SHEN yearly progression and the daily movements of the Personal Spirit (REN SHEN) are of primary importance. Since the first governs an entire lunar year it is easy to remember. Since the second is as easy to track as knowing which day of the lunar month it is, i.e. in traditional Chinese terms, knowing the day's date, this likewise is easy to remember. At the most this would only rule out two areas of the body available for treatment at any given time. Since there is usually more than one group of points capable of catalyzing a certain effect in the organism, avoidance of two, easy to calculate and remember body parts does not seem onerous. And in any case, the DA CHENG states that in the event of an acute illness all methods of proscription are to be disregarded. In other words, the proscriptions are only additional refinements in the treatment of chronic illnesses over a long period of time. They are not applicable or necessary to follow in the case of acute or life-threatening illnesses or accidents. Therefore, even if the ankle is prohibited to acupuncture on a certain day, if a patient comes in with a sprained ankle it is not considered inappropriate to needle it. In that case, acupuncture treatment is indicated on that area to redress the negative and considerably more deleterious effects of the injury itself.

In order for contemporary practitioners to recognize the value of considering these astrological proscriptions we must first understand what may happen if we disregard them. This is no easy matter to state succinctly since the DA CHENG does not spell this out in great detail. As stated above in discussing the JIU GONG KAO SHEN JIN JI or Nine House KAO SHEN Contraindications, the DA CHENG says that even light erroneous treatment may cause ulceration , presumably at the site of insertion, whereas heavy erroneous treatment may cause death. Ulceration due to infection suggests that the treatment dispersed the ZHENG or Righteous Qi in the area and allowed the penetration or accumulation of Evil Qi. Since the ZHENG QI is made up of a number of subcategories of energy, there are a number of possible scenarios explaining this in any given patient depending upon their constitution and condition at the time of treatment.

Peng Rong-chen, in "Exploration on Chrono-Acupuncture based on the Relationship of Nine Palace Chart and Bioclock", discusses astrological proscriptions to acupuncture under three categories. The first category is proscriptions based on the solar cycle, i.e. the seasons. Citing Chapter 26 of the SU WEN quoted above, Peng states that if one needles contrary to the seasonal ebb and flow of Qi and Blood one can disperse the Qi inappropriately, cause it to stagnate, or cause it to rebel perversely upward. The second category is based on the phases of the Moon on which the thirty day cycles are in turn based. Peng writes: "When the moon grows, the energy and the blood also begin to grow, so in administering acupuncture treatment stress must be laid on the promotion of its growth. If sedation is administered, it will go against the law of the universe that may cause injury of blood and energy. When the moon is full, the blood and energy has reached its zenith of abundance, so it is appropriate to make the blood and energy disperse. If tonification is further administered, it will still go against the law of the universe and that may give rise to the retaining of the blood and energy in the reticular meridians. When the moon is crescent, it is the time of wanting blood and energy, one must nurse his energy and should not go against the law of the universe to administer acupuncture treatment. This is to avoid the disturbance of the change of Yin and Yang energies." [17]

Peng's third category is the most interesting and the one which requires the most research and discussion. Peng states: "The human energy is in correspondence with the energies of Heaven and Earth. So in administering treatment, one must pay attention to the site where the human energy concentrates so as not to go against the law of universe genuinely."[18] Peng then goes on to give yet another set of proscriptions from the chapter on "The Yin Yang Meaning of the Sun and Moon" from the LING SHU: "In (the first, second, and third lunar months) the human energy is at the left side of the body, so no acupuncture treatment should be administered to the three Foot Yang meridians on the left lateral. In (the fourth, fifth, and sixth lunar months), the human energy is at the right side of the body, so no acupuncture treatment should be applied to the three Foot Yang meridians of the right lateral. In (the seventh, eighth, and nineth lunar months), the human energy still remains at the right side, so no acupuncture treatment should be given to the three Foot Yin meridians at the right lateral. In (the tenth, eleventh, and twelfth lunar months), the human energy goes back to the left side again, so no acupuncture treatment should be given to the three Foot Yin meridians at the left lateral."[19] In discussing the first two categories of proscriptions, Peng gives specific, easily understood, and theoretically logical examples of the physiologic harm intemperate acupuncture can cause. But in discussing the last category, Peng merely says the "human energy" may be injured. According to the table of proscriptions used to illustrate this third category, the "human energy" may be injured in a certain place at a certain time because it circulates in a definite pattern throughout the body and one runs the risk of harming it if one needles the site where it is currently residing.

The idea that some energy or energies circulate through the body according to various temporal cycles is implied in the DA CHENG as well. However, in the DA CHENG what is implied to circulate are various SHEN or spirits. In the Nine House KAO SHEN Contraindications, it is the KAO SHEN which resides in the various parts of the body during successive years and which may be harmed by inappropriate acupuncture. In the Personal Spirit of the Four Seasons Contraindications it is the Seasonal Personal Spirit which circulates and may be injured. In the Daily Movements of the Personal Spirit Contraindications found in both the DA CHENG and the much earlier HUANG TI MING TANG JIU JING, it is the Daily Personal Spirit which circulates and may be injured.

In contemporary Traditional Chinese Medicine, the SHEN or Spirit is usually discussed as a more or less discrete energy. Patients either have good Spirit which indicates a favorable prognosis or they have weak Spirit which indicates an unfavorable prognosis. This use of the term is similar to saying a race horse has spirit or is spirited. In addition, a patient's SHEN, which is said to reside in the Heart and is nurtured by the Blood, may become agitated or deranged due to Blood Deficiency, Heat, or Obstruction due to Phlegm. Nowhere in the modern literature is there any discussion of a temporal circuit of the body of this SHEN or Spirit since this would imply the existence of a transcendent, nonmaterialistic, and truely spiritual entity or entities residing in the body. This is something Confucian or JU YI medicine has not been wont to do since at least the rise of the HAN XUE PAI or Return to Han movement. This insistence that there is no transcendent aspect of the individual within the human organism has been adopted and dogmatised by the Communists since it would otherwise allow for a number of religious implications.

However, as Paul Unschuld ably points out in MEDICINE IN CHINA: A HISTORY OF IDEAS, Chinese medicine is not a single monolithic orthodoxy but rather a collection of various, sometimes even contradictory theories about the nature, cause, and treatment of illness.[20] The so-called Traditional Chinese Medicine endorsed and supported by the current regime in the Peoples' Republic of China is only one specific style or theory of Chinese medicine. This style of Chinese medicine has been chosen for governmental propagation since it can be understood and taught from a quasi-materialist point of view. The word SHEN as interpreted by Confucianists and their Communist successors has been given a non-religious meaning. However, I think it is safe to say that to the majority of Chinese over the last three millenia, the word SHEN has had distinctly and primarily religious connotations. SHEN is not only a philosophical or psychophysical abstraction. It also means spirit in the sense of an independent being existing on a non-material level. A DICTIONARY OF CHINESE BUDDHIST TERMS defines SHEN not only as a person's Spirit but also as a spirit.[21] This word also appears as part of the name of a large number of identifiable spirits in Chinese Buddhist demonology: SHIH ER SHEN (the Twelve Spirits associated with the Terrestial Branches and who are attendants of the Medicine Buddha), DA SHEN WANG (Mahakala, a fierce guardian spirit), LIU DA SHEN (the Six Great Spirits of the Six Elements, i.e. Earth, Water, Fire, Air, Space, and Mind), HUO SHEN (the 44 Fire Spirits), DI SHEN (Earth spirits in general and/or specifically Prthivi), XIANG SHEN (Gandharvas), KUEI SHEN (ghosts and spirits, including the spirits of the dead together with demons and the Eight Classes of spirits), MING SHEN (devas of a benevolent nature), etc., etc. Based on a comparison of spirit names appearing in A DICTIONARY OF CHINESE BUDDHIST TERMS, spirits whose names include the word SHEN tend to be associated with nature animistically. Whereas spirits whose names include the word TIAN (Heaven) tend to be dieties or gods, such as DA TIAN (Shiva).

In my essay on Tibetan moxabustion included in this volume there are similar prohibitions against the use of moxa at certain points at certain times. Many of these prohibitions are based on similar cycles of time as are the Chinese, such as a nine year cycle, the lunar day cycle, and the Terrestial Branches hourly cycle, although the actual proscribed locations are not the same. The Tibetan concept of what circulates through these cycles is the LA. This is defined as a person's life-force. The LA-NAY is the place or location at which the LA resides. A person can also have a LA associated with a place or object outside of themself, such as a rock, tree, or gemstone. A family, clan, or country can also have a communal LA residing in, for instance, a lake as does the national LA of Tibet. If this LA is harmed, it can cause a weakening and disease in either the individual or the group. If the LA is destroyed or departs from its residence, death may ensue. Dr. Trogawa Rinpoche has said that injury at the LA-NAY causes an inordinately strong reaction, including infection and ulceration. This is identical to the result of injuring the KAO SHEN given in the DA CHENG.

According to Tibetan medicine, if the LA is injured or has been forced out of its residence, it can be treated by ritual magic. In other words, it can be communicated with through liturgy and mantra. This implies that the LA is a type of SHEN or spirit. In fact, in Tibetan medicine there are possited a number of spirits residing in the body which can have an effect on the individual's health and well-being. These include the LUNG-LHA (Wind or Pranic spirit), WANG-LHA (personal power spirit), KYE-LHA (Birth spirit, i.e. personal guardian spirit),

PHO-LHA and MO-LHA (male and female personal spirits), and LU-LHA (Body spirit). In the Tibetan moxabustion essay there are descriptions of the deleterious effects of harming inadvertently through erroneous treatment any of the places of residence of these spirits comprising the individual's psychophysical organism. The Tibetan word LHA which means god or spirit corresponds directly with the Chinese word SHEN.

The implication is that some Chinese physicians have seen the body as being inhabited by a number of spirits which circulate through the body according to definite cycles. Whether these "spirits" are independent beings or are personifications and deifications of our psychophysical constituents is an interesting question. This question cannot, however, be answered succinctly since it involves a number of ontological and epistemological issues of great complexity. In fact, this question has to do with the limitations of language and rational thought. Such considerations are beyond the scope of this essay. However, such a belief in guardian or personal spirits would logically not be endorsed by the conservative Confucian nor the contemporary Communist medical tradition. But, just because one medical lineage has not accepted the existence of such personal spirits for philosophical reasons does not mean that such spirits do not exist nor that their manipulation is not clinically valuable or effective. All it means is that one group of Chinese doctors has seen fit not to incorporate this belief into their practice for largely non-medical reasons.[22] Since this group has become since the Communist revolution the dominant and state-endorsed version of Chinese medicine practiced in mainland China, it is not hard to understand why there is little mention of this belief and the medical practices based on it. However, Tibetan medicine has incorporated this notion into its orthodox body of knowledge and practice and its utility and truth have been verified during hundreds of years of clinical experience.

Historically it is probable that Tibetan and Chinese medical beliefs regarding the LA and SHEN stem from a common source. In the Tang dynasty when such astrological considerations first seem to have gained a prominent place in Chinese medicine, there was a great deal of cultural exchange between Tibet and China. Tibetan nobility regularly went to China to receive their education in medicine and astrology.[23] Later on, in the Yuan and Ming dynasties, a succession of Tibetan Lamas were appointed as tutors to the Imperial court. This included their sending and administering medicines to the Emperor. Therefore the Tibetans could have gotten the idea of the circulation of the LA from the Chinese during the Tang or the Chinese could have in turn been influenced by the Tibetans during the Yuan and Ming when Dou Han-jing and Yang Ji-zhou were writing. It is interesting to note that the pre-Buddhist or Bon-po Tibetan word for a sorcerer capable of manipulating the spirit world is likewise SHEN. However, who got what from whom and when are questions beyond my expertise.

There have always been Chinese doctors who not only beleived in and used the theories of correspondence of Yin and Yang and the Five Elements but also believed in and used spiritual interventions as well. Sun Si-miao is a good example of such a doctor. Sun was considered an expert in the I JING and Yin-Yang theory as well having comprehensive knowledge of both the acupuncture and pharmocological lore of his day. He wrote treatises on herbal medicine (CHIEN JIN FANG) and on ritual and incantory magic (CHIN JING, THE CLASSIC OF INTERDICTIONS).[24] Sun was also considered a LING YI or professional, clinically experienced doctor and he numbered himself amongst the DA YI or superior practitioner of his time.[25] By denying the validity of medical intervention on spiritual levels, conservative Confucianists and Communists alike have cut themselves off from both the very source of life and from a truly holistic medicine. For no medicine which denies the transcendent nature of human life can adequately minister to the whole person. Despite Communist repression, the temples and churches of China are full to overflowing. Nor is it hard to understand why American churches, synagogues, and temples are once again flourishing. A medicine which does not adequately address the spiritual needs of spiritual beings cannot provide a complete and comprehensive treatment for the alleviation of suffering.

Because China has been and is such a huge and heterogeneous country, Chinese medicine is, unlike Tibetan medicine, heterogeneous. It is my belief that the secular and materialist version of Chinese medicine which currently proports to be the true orthodoxy of this art is inadequate conceptually to treat the whole person on all levels including the Spirit. It is also my belief that, as we plunge ever deeper into the morass of problems created because of materialist-inspired technological solutions to essential existential, spiritual problems, the necessary corrective is renewed emphasis on the spiritual. Prohibitions regarding Closed points in acupuncture are, it seems to me, based on a spiritual appreciation of the psychophysical makeup of the human organism. Consideration of and research into these prohibitions draws attention to both the limitations of the TCM party line and the necessity of nurturing and protecting the Spirit of our patients. As such, I beleive they can be clincally valuable and spiritually instructive.

ENDNOTES

1 I CHING OR BOOK OF CHANGES, trans. Richard Willhelm & Cary Baynes, Princeton University Press, Princeton, 1967, p. 713

2 Willhelm, Helmut, HEAVEN, EARTH AND MAN IN THE BOOK OF CHANGES, University of Washington Press, Seattle & London, 1977, p. 16-7

3 Lu Gwei-djen & Needham, Joseph, CELESTIAL LANCETS, Cambridge University Press, Cambridge & London, 1980, p. 140

4 Needham, Joseph & Wang Ling, SCIENCE AND CIVILIZATION IN CHINA, Cambridge University Press, Cambridge & London, 1956, Vol. 3, p. 396-8

5 Porkert, Manfred, THE THEORETICAL FOUNDATIONS OF CHINESE MEDICINE MIT Press, Cambridge, MA & London, 1982, p. 60-103

6 Yang Ji-zhou, ZHEN JIU DA CHENG, Peoples Health Press, Beijing, 1973, p. 141-2

7 Tou Gui-fang, HUANG TI MING TANG JIU JING, Peoples Health Press, Beijing 1983, p. 4

8 Yang, op. cit., p. 143

9 Ibid., p. 144

10 HUANG TI NEI JING TAI SU; HUANG TI NEI JING SU WEN, Chap. 26; & Huang Pu-mi's JIA YI JING, Chap. 5

11 Yang, op. cit., p. 143

12 Ibid., p. 144

13 Ibid., p. 143

14 Ibid., p. 144

15 Ibid., p. 143

16 Tou, op. cit., p. 4

17 Peng Rong-chen, "Exploration on Chrono-Acupuncture based on the Relationship of Nine-Palace Chart and Bioclock", SELECTIONS FROM SHANGHAI JOURNAL OF ACUPUNCTURE AND MOXIBUSTION, 1982-1984, Shanghai Institute of Acupuncture and Meridians, Shanghai, 1984, p. 209

18 Ibid., p. 209

19 Ibid., p. 209

[20] Unschuld, Paul U., MEDICINE IN CHINA: A HISTORY OF IDEAS, University of CA Press, Berkeley, LA, & London, 1985

[21] Soothill, William E. & Hodous, Lewis, A DICTIONARY OF CHINESE BUDDHIST TERMS, Motilal Banarsidas, Delhi, Varanasi, & Patna, 1977, p. 334

[22] Unschuld, op. cit., p. 61-6

[23] Dowman, Keith, SKY DANCER, Routledge & Kegan Paul, London, etc., 1984, p. 332

[24] Unschuld, op. cit., p. 303-4

[25] Unschuld, Paul U., MEDICAL ETHICS IN IMPERIAL CHINA, University of CA Press, Berkeley, LA, & London, 1979, p. 25-6

THE EIGHT EXTRA MERIDIANS

Their Clinical Use according to the ZHEN JIU DA CHENG

According to Dou Han-jing of the Yuan dynasty, "The eight crossing points of the extra channels are the essentials of acupuncture."[1] In the Ming dynasty, Li Shi-zhen again emphasized the importance of the eight Extraordinary vessels and their command or crossing points in clinical practice when he stated that any doctor not employing the eight Extraordinary vessels is not practicing the highest form of medicine.[2] Li Yan, a famous clinican also of the Ming, in his GUIDE-BOOK TO MEDICINE, further elucidated their importance in the following succinct summation: "In the eight therapeutics, the eight points of (the) extra channels are of prime importance. They are the common pool of the twelve regular channels ... There are three hundred sixty points on the whole body, controlled by sixty-six points on the limbs, which in turn are controlled by eight points."[3] It is clear from the above statements by eminent classical doctors that the eight Extraordinary vessels and their command points were regarded as being of key importance to the practice of acupuncture. In fact, Li Yan held them to be the eight most important points in the body. However, in contemporary TCM acupuncture these eight points have not retained the stature they once held.

In part, the preeminence of the eight command points of the Extraordinary vessels has been obscured by the wide disparity of opinion held upon their proper usage. Some practitioners in the PRC today, for instance, may simply needle a single point on the REN MAI and declare the REN MAI activated, thus invoking the efficacy of its being an Extraordinary vessel. Others may needle only one of the paired command points without employing the other, for instance needling GONG SUN (Sp 4), the command point of the CHONG MO, without simultaneously needling NEI GUAN (Per 6), its paired point on the YIN WEI MO. Some European schools, as exemplified by the techniques given in Woolerton and Mc Lean's ACUPUNCTURE ENERGY IN HEALTH & DISEASE, give detailed specific needling sequences for accessing these vessels.[4] Different but no less detailed and specific sequences, even employing needles made out of various specific metals, have been created by contemporary Japanese practitioners such as Yoshio

Manaka. Then there's the LING GUEI PA FA method of using the eight command points based on certain of these being open at specific astrologically determined times. All these various techniques and opinions have, to some extent, blunted the enthusiasm and faith of many modern acupuncturists in the special efficacy of these points. As some have reasoned, if these points are so special, it seems logical that their use might likewise require some special technique. However, can all these techniques be equally valid? Although doubt sown by the existence of differences of opinion in the literature fails to take into account some of the deeper questions about the nature of acupuncture as a healing modality, it does suggest that more attention be paid to the usage of these points and vessels.

The locus classicus of the eight command points of the Extraordinary vessels being grouped into four pairs is Dou Han-jing's GUIDE TO ACUPUNCTURE.[5] Although the NEI JING and NAN JING speak of the eight Extraordinary vessels, these command points are not listed as such in such early classics. Therefore these eight points are also sometimes refered to as "Dou's Eight Points" similar to "Ma's Twelve Stars". An article authored anonymously under the auspices of the Beijing College of TCM appearing in MEDECINE TRADITIONELLE CHINOISES ET ACUPUNCTURE states that although the eight command points of the Extraordinary vessels may be needled singly and/or in combination with other adjunct points, their most effective use is when they are used as pairs.[6] Of the four pairs, one command point on the upper extremities is paired with another on the lower extremities. "By combined use of the hand and foot channels, balance of Qi in the channels can be achieved through mutual affection between the upper and lower. This is very advantageous to the adjustment and execution of visceral functions."[7] In Dou's GUIDE TO ACUPUNCTURE, two hundred thirteen syndromes are listed as indications for the eight Extraordinary vessel command points.[8] According to Dou, "all these syndromes can be successfully treated by first deciding which regular and extra channels are involved with respect to the presenting symptoms as well as the causative 'evil', and then needling the point (on the regular channel) that communicates with the particular extra channel."[9]

This method of Dou's was later systematized by Yang Ji-zhou in THE GREAT COMPENDIUM OF ACUPUNCTURE & MOXABUSTION (ZHEN JIU DA CHENG) of the Ming dynasty. Yang put this material into verse so that it could be more easily memorized. This use of the eight Extraordinary vessels is covered in the 5th CHUAN of the ZHEN JIU DA CHENG entitled "Chart of the Eight Vessels as used in conjunction with symptomatic points". The ZHEN JIU DA CHENG is widely held to be the pinnacle of classical Chinese acupuncture literature.[10] Presented below is a translation of this section of the DA CHENG by Chip Chace. It is offered not in the belief that this is the only valid usage of the eight Extraordinary vessels. Any method's validity ultimately must depend upon its clinical results. It is presented rather as one of the most respected classical dissertations on this topic so that contemporary acupuncturists may 1) have access to these techniques and 2) may also upgrade their scholarship. Before one can judge the probable worth of a technique or theory presented as traditional Chinese, one should know where and when it originated. In that way one can chart the history of such a technique or theory over a period of time and see whether or not its claims have been substantiated in practice. Without such scholarship, one must test each theory or technique afresh with equal attention. This is equivalent to reinventing the wheel and wastes time duplicating in the dark what generations of practitioners may already have ascertained.

CHUAN # 5

"Chart of the Eight Vessels as used in conjunction with symptomatic points"

From Yang Ji-zhou's **ZHEN JIU DA CHENG**

CHONG MAI

GONG SUN (Sp 4) lies bilaterally on the Spleen Channel. It is located one CUN behind the base joint of the large toe in a hollow and is needled to a depth of one CUN. It governs diseases of the Heart, abdomen, and five solid organs. NEI GUAN (Per 6) is tis corresponding point of influence.

Symptomology (According to Xi Jiang-yue): GONG SUN treats the nine types of Heart disorders, knotted chest[11], stagnant and upset Stomach, accumulations of food and drink in the Stomach, intestinal rumbling, diaphragmatic disturbances, umbilical pain, abdominal soreness, distention of the sides, intestinal wind, malaria, acute Heart pain, retained placenta, confusion, and diarrhea. GONG SUN will get an immediate response.

When treating the following symptoms, use GONG SUN first as the controller; then employ the other appropriate points (according to Xu)[12].

The nine kinds of Heart pain[13], and all types of Stagnant Cold: DA LING (Per 7), ZHONG WAN (CV 12), YIN BAI (Sp 1)

Phlegm in the diaphragm causing stuffiness and oppression (and) ill-defined pain in the chest: LAO GONG (Per 8), SHAN ZHONG (CV 17), JIAN SHI (Per 5)

Stagnancy of the diaphragm, the five kinds of choking[14], (and for) food and drink (that) will not descend: SHAN ZHONG, ZU SAN LI (St 36), TAI BAI (Sp 3)

Abdominal distention and fullness, particularly around the umbilicus, and indigestion: TIAN SHU (St 25), SHUI FEN (CV 9), NEI TING (St 44)

Intercostal pain with difficulty in standing: ZHI GOU (TH 6), YANG LING QUAN (GB 34), ZHANG MEN (Liv 13)

Incessant diarrhea with tenesmus: XIA WAN (CV 10), TIAN SHU, ZHAO HAI (Ki 6)

Stabbing chest pain and inability to enjoy thing: NEI TING, DA LING, YU ZHONG (Ki 26)

Bilateral distention and fullness of the costal region[15] due to Qi attacking causing soreness and pain: JUE GU (GB 39), ZHANG MEN, YANG LING QUAN

Feeling out of sorts with a sense of epigastric fullness, FAN WEI[16], vomiting food: ZHONG WAN, TAI BAI, ZHONG KUEI (LI 5)

Stagnancy of Phlegm in the Stomach, vomiting of clear fluid: JU QUE (CV 14),

ZHONG WAN, LI DUI (St 45)

Stagnancy of food in the Stomach characterized by ceaseless stabbing pain and soreness: ZHONG WAN, ZU SAN LI, JIE XI (St 41)

Vomiting of Phlegm with intractable dizziness: SHAN ZHONG, ZHONG KUEI, FENG LONG

Cardiac malaria[17] characterized by palpitations: SHEN MEN (Ht 7), XIN SHU (Bl 15), BAI LAO (GV 14)

Splenic malaria characterized by chillophobia and abdominal pain: SHANG QUI (Sp 5), PI SHU (Bl 20), ZU SAN LI

Hepatic malaria characterized by a greenish facial hue; there will also be fever and chills: ZHONG FENG (Liv 4), GAN SHU (Bl 18), JUE GU

Pulmonary malaria resulting in a sense of cold in the Heart and palpitations: LIE QUE (Lu 7), FEI SHU (Bl 13), HE GU (LI 4)

Renal malaria causing a person to be bathed in fever[18] with lumbar and spinal stiffness and pain: DA ZHONG (Ki 4), SHEN SHU (Bl 23), SHEN MAI (Bl 62)

Acute malaria characterized by unrelenting fever: JIAN SHI, BAI LAO, JUE GU[19a]

Intermittent fever, first chills, then fever: HOU XI (SI 3), QU CHI (LI 11), LAO GONG

Intermittent fever, first fever, then chills: QU CHI, BAI LAO, DA SHU (Bl 11), JUE GU

Intermittent fever with pain in the Heart and chest: NEI GUAN, SHANG WAN (CV 13), DA LING

Intermittent fever with headache, dizziness, and incessant vomiting of Phlegm: HE GU, ZHONG WAN, LIE QUE

Intermittent fever with arthralgia: PO HU (Bl 42), BAI LAO, RANG GU (Ki 2)

Intermittent fever with incessant thirst: GUAN CHONG (TH 1), REN ZHONG (GV 26), JIAN SHI

Gastric malaria causing the patient to have a good appetite but be unable to eat: LI DUI, WEI SHU (Bl 21), DA DU (Sp 2)

Biliary malaria causing the patient to experience chiilophobia and palpitations as well as restless sleep: LIN QI (GB 41), DAN SHU (Bl 19), QI MEN (Liv 14)

Jaundice characterized by yellowness of the skin of the entire body as well as the face and eyes; the urine is particularly yellow: PI SHU, YIN BAI, BAI LAO, ZHI YANG (GV 9), ZU SAN LI, WAN GU (SI 4), YIN GU (Ki 10)

Jaundice characterized by swelling of the four limbs; perspiration stains the clothes: ZHI YANG, BAI LAO, WAN GU, ZHONG WAN, ZU SAN LI

Grain jaundice whose symptoms are dizziness after eating, a sense of obstruction and pain in the Heart, an the jaundicing of the entire body: WEI SHU, NEI TING, ZHI YANG, ZU SAN LI, WAN GU, YIN GU

Wine jaundice characterized by yellowness of the entire body including the eyes, Heart pain, a rash which develops on the face, and reddish yellow urine: DAN SHU, ZHI YANG, WEI ZHONG (Bl 40), WAN GU

Feminine consumptive jaundice characterized by yellowness of the entire body including the eyes with fever and chills and difficult urination: GUAN YUAN (CV 4), SHEN SHU, ZHI YANG, RANG GU

Yang's Symptomology:

Irregular menstruation: GUAN YUAN, QI HAI (CV 6), TIAN SHU, SAN YIN JIAO (Sp 6)

Fullness and pain in the chest: LAO GONG, TONG LI (Ht 5), DA LING, SHAN ZHONG

Phlegm Heat knots the chest: LIE QUE, DA LING, YONG QUAN (Ki 1)

Wind pain in the four limbs: QU CHI, FENG SHI (GB 31), wai guan 9th 5), YANG LING QUAN (GB 34), SAN YIN JIAO, SHOU SAN LI (LI 10)

Obstruction in the throat: SHAO SHANG (Lu 11), FENG CHI (GB 20), JIA CHE (St 6)

YIN WEI MAI

NEI GUAN lies bilaterally on the Pericardium Channel. It is locate two CUN above the palm between the two tendons when a fist is formed. It is needled to a depth of one CUN, two FEN. This point governs diseases of the Heart, Gallbladder, Spleen, and Stomach. GONG SUN is its corresponding point of influence.

Symptomology (according to Xi Jiang-yue): NEI GUAN treats epigastric fullness, distention of the Heart and chest, intestinal rumbling, diarrhea, rectal prolapse, difficulty in passing food below the diaphragm, and injury from excessive consumption of alcohol, a stagnant lump fixed in the side causing one to grasp it, soreness in the sides and Heart pain in women, knotted chest and an internal uneasiness which is difficult to bear, knotted chest due to an unresolved injury due to Cold. NEI GUAN used alone can treat these symptoms. When treating the following symptoms, use NEI GUAN first as the controlling point and then employ the other appropriate points (according to Xu).

Epigastric fullness without a tumor; the gastric cavity suffers injury caused by Cold: ZHONG WAN, DA LING, ZU SAN LI, SHAN ZHONG

Distention and fullness in the Middle Burner and bilateral stabbing pains in the sides: ZHI GOU, ZHANG MEN, SHAN ZHONG

Insufficiency of Stomach/Spleen Qi and distention and fullness of the subcardiac region: TAI BAI, ZU SAN LI, QI HAI, SHUI FEN

Coldness and insufficiency of the Stomach/Spleen with incessant vomiting: NEI TING, ZHONG WAN, QI HAI, GONG SUN

Hypochondral soreness and a stabbing pain in the upper abdomen: QI HAI, XING JIAN (Liv 2), YANG LING QUAN

Intractable fixed tumor; pain and oppression in the Heart: DA LING, ZHONG WAN, SAN YIN JIAO

Food obstruction of the bowels which does not disperse; the patient gradually becomes emaciated: WAN GU, PI SHU, GONG SUN

Stagnant food, XUE JIA[19b], indistinct pain in the abdomen: WEI SHU, XING JIAN, QI HAI

The five Stagnant Qi lumps and Blood Stagnation: GE SHU (Bl 17), GAN SHU, DA DUN (Liv 1), ZHAO HAI (Ki 6)

Insufficiency and chill of the ZANG FU and bilateral pain and soreness in the sides: ZHI GOU, TONG LI, ZHANG MEN, YANG LING QUAN

Wind Obstruction and Qi Stagnation with stabbing pain in the subcardiac region: FENG MEN (Bl 12), SHAN ZHONG, LAO GONG, ZU SAN LI

Insufficiency and chill in the Large Intestine with anal prolapse: BAI HUI (GV 20), MING MEN (GV 4), CHANG JIANG (GV 1), CHENG SHAN (Bl 57)

Difficult defecation the exertion of which causes prolapse: ZHAO HAI, BAI HUI, ZHI GOU

Visceral toxicity with pain and swelling[20], incessant hemafecia: CHENG SHAN, GAN SHU, GE SHU, CHANG JIANG

Five types of acute hemorrhoids causing incessant pain: HE YANG (Bl 55), CHANG JIANG, CHENG SHAN

Five types of convulsions with spittle coming from the mouth: HOU XI (SI 3), SHEN MEN, XIN SHU, KUEI YAN (Sp 1)

Dementia and incessant weeping with grief: TONG LI, HOU XI, SHEN MEN, DA ZHONG

Fearfulness which leads to madness; one cannot tell friends from enemies: SHAO ZHONG (Ht 9), XIN SHU, ZHONG WAN, SHI XUAN (Extra points)

Forgetfullness and muddled speech: xin shu, tong li, shao zhong

Insufficiency of Heart Qi where there may be laughing or singing: LING DAO (Ht 4), XIN SHU, TONG LI

Palpitations and raving: SHAO HAI (Ht 3), SHAO FU (Ht 8), XIN SHU, HOU XI

Heart Deficiency and upset; the mind lacks serenity: RU GEN (St 18), TONG LI, DAN SHU, XIN SHU

Palpitations and stroke with unconsciousness: ZHONG CHONG (Per 9), BAI HUI, DA DUN

All-pervading Heart Insufficiency and palpitations: YIN XI (Ht 6), XIN SHU, TONG LI

Heart Insufficiency and chill in the Gallbladder characterized by unsteadiness of the four limbs: DAN SHU, TONG LI, LIN QI

DU MAI

HOU XI lies bilaterally on the Small Intestine Channel. It is located on the outside of the small finger in a hollow next to the metacarpalphalangeal joint when a fist is made and is needled to a depth of one CUN. HOU XI controls disorders of the head, face, and neck. SHEN MAI (Bl 62) is its corresponding point of influence.

Symptomology (according to Xi Jiang-yue): Rigidity and contracture in the hands and feet, trembling and shaking, stroke with aphonia and convulsions, headache, swollen eyes, constant lacrimation; pain in the leg, knee, spine, and lumbar regions; stiff neck due to unresolved injury by Cold; swollen jaws and gums, sore throat, numbness in the hands and feet and tetany; night sweats. Needle HOU XI first. When treating the following symptoms, needle HOU XI first as the controlling point and then employ the other points (according to Xu).

Rapid contracture of the hands and feet with difficulty in bending and stretching: ZU SAN LI, QU CHI, CHI ZE (Lu 5), HE GU, XING JIAN, YANG LING QUAN

Tremors of the hands and feet making it impossible to hold onto things: YANG XI (LI 5), QU CHI, WAN GU, TAI CHONG (Liv 3), JUE GU, GONG SUN, YANG LING QUAN

Stiffness and pain in the neck making it impossible to look behind: CHENG JIANG (CV 24), FENG CHI, FENG FU (GV 16)

Swelling, redness, and pain in the cheeks: DA YING (St 5), JAI CHE, HE GU

Obstruction in the throat where even a droplet of water cannot be swallowed: DA LING, SHANG YANG (LI 7), ZHAO HAI, SHI XUAN

Double Moth Wind[21] with stricture of the throat: SHAO SHANG, JIN JIN (Extra point), YU YE (Extra point), SHI XUAN

Simple Moth Wind; throat is swollen and painful: GUAN CHONG, TIAN TU (CV 22), HE GU

Head Wind[22] which is located in the center of the head as well as temporally, the corners of the forehead being particularly painful: LIE QUE, HE GU, TAI YANG (purple vein), Head LIN QI (GB 15), SI ZHU KUNG (TH 23)

Incessant pain at the corners of the eyebrows: ZAN ZHU (Bl 2), YANG BAI (GB 14), YIN TANG (Extra point), HE GU, TOU WEI (St 8)

Head and eyes are cloudy and befuddled with pain at TAI YANG: HE GU, the purple vein at TAI YANG, TOU WEI

Spasm of the head and neck which leads to pain in the shoulder and spine: CHENG JIANG, BAI HUI, JIAN JING (GB 21), ZHONG ZHU (TH 3)

Drunken Head Wind with incessant vomiting and aversion to hearing peoples' voices: YONG QUAN, LIE QUE, BAI LAO, HE GU

Red, swollen eyes with incessant lacrimation due to an insulting Wind: ZAN ZHU, HE GU, XIAO QU KUNG (Extra point),[23] Head LIN QI

Tetanus; a tic develops due to one's lifestyle; there is a strong fever in the entire body: DA DUN, HE GU, XING JIAN, SHI QUAN, & bleed the vein at TAI YANG

Yang's Symptomology:

Cough due to Cold Phlegm: LIE QUE, YONG QUAN, SHEN MAI, TIAN TU, SI ZHU KUNG

Dizziness of the head and eyes: FENG CHI, MING MEN, HE GU

Stiff neck: CHENG JIANG, FENG FU, FENG CHI, HE GU

Toothache: LIE QUE, REN ZHONG, JIA CHE, TAI XI (Ki 3), TAI YUAN (Lu

9), HE GU

Deafness: TING HUI (GB 2), SHANG YANG (LI 1), SHAO CHONG, ZHONG CHONG

Tetanus: CHENG JIANG, HE GU, BA XIE (Extra points), HOU XI, WAI GUAN, SI QUAN (Liv 3), HE GU

YANG QIAO MAI

SHEN MAI is situated bilaterally on the Urinary Bladder Channel. It is located on the outside of the ankle in a hollow at the juncture of the red and white flesh and is needled to a depth of one CUN. SHEN MAI controls WIND EVIL in the four limbs as well as diseases such as carbuncles. HOU XI is tis corresponding point of influence.

Symptomology (according to Xi Jiang-yue): Stiffness of the spine and lumbar region, swelling of the legs, amenophobia, spontaneous perspiration and headache, thundering headache[24a], red eyes, pain at the corner of the eyebrows; numbess and contracture of the hands and feet and coldness of the arms; blowing and sucking deafness, epistaxis, arthralgia, swelling and distention of the entire body, and the entire body drenched in sweat. When treating the following symptoms, use SHEN MAI first as the controlling point and then employ other appropriate points (according to Xu).

Stiffness in the spine and lumbar region so severe that one cannot lift or bend one's head: YAO SHU (GV 3), GAO HUANG SHU (Bl 43), WEI ZHONG (bleed purple vein)

Arthralgia in the four limbs and soreness in the legs and lumbar region due to strain: JIAN YU (LI 15), QU CHI, KUN LUN (Bl 60), YANG LING QUAN

Unconsciousness due to stroke: ZHONG CHONG, BAI HUI, DA DUN, YIN TANG, HE GU

Aphonia due to stroke: SHAO SHANG, REN ZHONG, SHAN ZHONG, HE GU, YA MEN (GV 15)

Stroke with partial paralysis: SHOU SAN LI, WAN GU, HE GU, JUE GU, XING JIAN, FENG SHI, SAN YIN JIAO

Stroke with hemiplegia and incessant pain and soreness: JUE GU, TAI YUAN, QU CHI, JIAN YU, ZU SAN LI, KUN LUN

Stroke with numbess and paralysis of the extremities: ZHOU LIAO (LI 12), SHANG LIAN (LI 9), YU JI (Lu 10), FENG SHI, XI QUAN (GB 33), SAN YIN JIAO

Stroke with itchiness of the hands and feet and inability to hold objects: NAO HUI (TH 13), WAN GU, HE GU, XING JIAN, FENG SHI, SAN YIN JIAO

Stroke with deviation of mouth and eyes (this condition being constant): REN ZHONG, HE GU, TAI YUAN, SHI XUAN, TONG ZI LIAO (GB 1), JIA CHE (needle one FEN, then needle towards DI CANG, St 4); if mouth is deviated to the right, then drain the left and vice versa. One may also moxa twenty times.

Stroke with opisthotonus and blindness: BAI HUI, BAI LAO, HE GU, QU CHI,

XING JIAN, SHI XUAN, YANG LING QUAN

Stroke with lockjaw and feeble, unintelligible speech: DI CANG (with strong stimulation), JIA CHE, REN ZHONG, HE GU

Soreness and pain in the neck, spine, and lumbar region: SHEN SHU, REN ZHONG, JIAN JING, WEI ZHONG

Lumbar pain with difficulty standing up: RANG GU, GAO HUANG SHU, WEI ZHONG, SHEN SHU

Sores on the back of the foot; this condition is known as a "carbuncle": NEI TING, XIA XI (GB 43), XING JIAN, WEI ZHONG

Sores on the back of the hand; this is known as carbuncle attached to the muscle: YE MEN (TH 2), ZHONG ZHU, HE GU, WAI GUAN

Sores on the arm and hand; this condition is known as an ulcer attached to the bone: TIAN FU (Lu 3), QU CHI, WEI ZHONG

Yang's Symptomology:

Ulcers on the back and shoulders: WEI ZHONG, XIA XI, SHI XUAN, QU CHI, YE MEN, NEI GUAN, WAI GUAN

Soreness of the entire body: TAI YUAN, ZU SAN LI, QU CHI

Injury to the neck or brain: BAI LAO, HE GU, SHEN MAI, CHIANG JIAN (GV 18), WEI ZHONG

Dull headache: SHEN MAI, JIN MEN (Bl 63), CHENG JIANG

Difficulty in rotating the neck: HOU XI, HE GU, CHENG JIANG

Sores on the upper lip (literally the mustache): TAI YUAN, SHEN MAI, TAI XI, HE GU, WAI GUAN

DAI MAI

LIN QI (GB 41) is situated bilaterally on the Gallbladder Channel. It is located one CUN distal to the juncture of the fourth and fifth metatrsal bones in a hollow and is needled to a depth of five FEN. In order to drain it, needle transversely along the skin one CUN. LIN QI treats disorders of the extremities and WAI GUAN is its corresponding point of influence.

Symptomology (according to Xi jiang-yue): Stroke causing immobility of the hands and feet, pain, numbness, fever and spasm, Head Wind and radiating pain and swelling of the neck and cheek, red, sore, and swollen eyes, as well as dizziness; toothache, deafness, swollen throat, and edema pruritus; pulled muscle and soreness in the legs. LIN QI proves effective when needled. When treating the following symptoms, needle LIN QI first as the controlling point; then employ the other points (according to Xu).

Chronic pain and swelling of the foot and ankle: XING JIAN, SHEN MAI

Paralysis of the hands and feet with inability to descriminate between itching and pain: TAI CHONG, QU CHI, DA LING, HE GU, ZU SAN LI, ZHONG ZHU

Pedal tremors and inability to walk: TAI CHONG, KUN LUN, YANG LING QUAN

Tremors of the hands and inability to grasp things: QU ZE (Per 3), WAN GU, HE GU, ZHONG ZHU

Spasms of the fingers and inabiltiy to grasp things: QU ZE, WAN GU, HE GU, ZHONG ZHU

Spasms of the toes and inability to flex the joints of the ten toes; curl the toes and burn young barley on the knuckles five times; (then needle): QI XU (GB 40), GONG SUN, YANG LING QUAN

Spasms of the fingers such that extending them causes pain and soreness; make a fist and burn young barley on the knuckles (the proximal interphalangeal joints) five times; (then needle): CHI ZE, YANG XI (LI 5), ZHONG ZHU

Heat in the soles of the feet; this is considered Damp Heat: YONG QUAN, JING QU (Bl 64), HE GU

Swelling and redness of the lateral malleolus; this is known as Wind boring into the ankles: KUN LUN, QI XU, ZHAO HAI

Sensation of heat on the instep and pain in the joints of the toes: CHANG YANG (St 42), XIA XI, Foot SHI XUAN (Extra points)

Sensation of heat in the hands and pain in the fingers: YANG CHI (TH 4), YE MEN, HE GU

Redness, swelling, and pain in the knees known as Crane's Knee Wind: XI QUAN (Liv 7), XING JIAN, FENG SHI, YANG LING QUAN

Painful wrist bones knwon as Wind surrounding the wrist: TAI YUAN, WAN GU, DA LING

Pain and soreness of the thighs and lumbar region known as Cold Hernia: WEI ZHONG, SAN YIN JIAO, WU SHU (GB 27)

Pain in the upper arm which radiates to the shoulder and spine: JIAN JING, QU CHI, ZHONG ZHU

Soreness and pain in the legs and thighs known as Leg-crossing Wind: HUAN TIAO (GB 30), WEI ZHONG, YANG LING QUAN

The extremities are sore and painful: JIAN JING, ZU SAN LI, QU CHI, WEI ZHONG, HE GU, XING JIAN, TIAN YING (the point will be tender; bleed it) 24b

The entire body itches: BAI HUI, BAI LAO, MING MEN, TAI YANG PURPLE vein, FENG SHI, JUE GU, SHUI FEN, QI HAI, XUE HAI (Sp 10), WEI ZHONG, QU CHI

Redness, swelling, stiffness, and pain in the neck: CHENG JIANG, FENG CHI, JIAN JING, FENG FU

Lumbar pain due to Kidney Deficiency with difficulty getting up and moving about: SHEN SHU, JI ZHONG (GV 6)

Acute lumbar pain wit difficulty standing up: JI ZHONG, SHEN SHU, YAO SHU (GV 2)

Lumbar pain due to Deficiency and Damp Obstruction where there is no strength in movement: JI ZHONG, YAO SHU, SHEN SHU, WEI ZHONG

Generalized Deficiency and weakness in the extremities: BAI LAO, XIN SHU, ZU SAN LI, GUAN YUAN, GAO HUANG SHU

A Qi lump causing stabbing pain in the sides due to Liver Qi Stagnation: ZHANG MEN, ZHI GOU, ZHONG WAN, DA LING, YANG LING QUAN

Yang's symptomology:

Spasms of the hands and feet: ZHONG ZHU, CHI ZE, JUE GU, BA XIE, YANG XI, YANG LING QUAN

"Labor pours into the four limbs": ZU SAN LI, WEI ZHONG, MING MEN, TIAN YING, QU CHI, WAI GUAN

Aches and pain in the knees and shins: XING JIAN, JUE GU, TAI CHONG, XI YAN (St 35), ZU SAN LI, YANG LING QUAN

Cold Obstruction pain in the legs: TAI CHONG, HE GU, JUE GU, FENG SHI, HUAN TIAO, SAN YIN JIAO

Pain and soreness in all the joints: HUN MEN (Bl 47), JUE GU, MING MEN, WAI GUAN

YANG WEI MAI

WAI GUAN is situated bilaterally on the Triple Heater Channel. It is located two CUN above the wrist on the back side of the palm in a hollow between the tendons with the hand bent and is needled to a depth of one CUN, two FEN. WAI GUAN treats Wind Cold in the channels and collaterals as well as skin diseases. LIN QI is its cooresponding point of influence.

Symptomology (according to Xi Jiang-yue): Soreness and swelling in the joints and limbs, cold knees, unresponsiveness of the forelimbs, Head Wind, pathogenic invasion of the medial and lateral aspect of the bones and the tendons of the back and the thighs, occipetal and superciliary head pain, hotness or numbness of the hands and feet, furtive perspiration, tetany, swollen eyes and bloodshot eyeballs, pathogenic injury due to Cold, spontaneous sweating and surface fever. (For all of the above) WAI GUAN alone is important for treatment. when treating the following symptoms, needle WAI GUAN first as the controlling point; then employ the other points (according to Xu).

Redness and swelling in the upper arm and shoulder as well as soreness and pain in the joints of the limbs: ZHOU LIAO (LI 12), JIAN LIAO (TH 14), WAN GU

Redness, sweeling, and pain of the medial malleolus known as Wind coils around the ankle: TAI XI, QI XU, LIN QI, KUN LUN

Pain in the finger joints such that thye cannot be extended: YANG GU (SI 5), WU HU (Extra point[25]), WAN GU, HE GU

Heat congests the Five Organs with incessant hematemesis; choose the SHU points of the Five Organs: XIN SHU, PI SHU, GAN SHU, SHEN SHU, GE SHU

Heat congests the Six Bowels with incessant hemorrhage; choose the six SHU points of the Bowels and additionally treat the Blood: XIAO CHANG SHU (Bl 27), DAN SHU, WEI SHU, DA CHANG SHU (Bl 25), PANG GUANG SHU (Bl 28), SAN JIAO SHU (Bl 22), GE SHU

Incessant nosebleed known as Blood running reckless: SHAO ZE, GE SHU, YONG QUAN

Hematemesis with dizziness and unconsciousness: GAN SHU, GE SHU, TONG LI, DA DUN

Reflux of Qi arising from Deficiency with incessant hematemesis: GAO HUANG SHU, GE SHU, DAN TIEN (CV 6), GAN SHU

Hematemesis and epistaxis where the Yang victimizes the Yin and Hot Blood runs reckless: ZHONG CHONG, GAN SHU, GE SHU, ZU SAN LI, SAN YIN JIAO

Cold Blood with vomiting where the Yin victimizes the Yang; this is known as vomiting Blood from the Heart and Lung Channels: SHAO SHANG, XIN SHU, SHEN MEN, FEI SHU (Bl 13), GE SHU, SAN YIN JIAO

Tongue stiffness and difficulty speaking with a white tongue fur: QUAN CHONG, ZHONG CHONG, CHENG JIANG

Tongue is thick and swollen; extreme Heat causes difficulty in speaking: SHI XUAN, HAI YUAN (Extra point[26]), JIN JIN, YU YE

Sores on the inside of the mouth known as Withering Groove Wind: DUI DUAN (GV 27), ZHI GOU, CHENG JIANG, SHI XUAN

Tongue which will not retract known as Yang rigidity: YONG QUAN, DUI DUAN, SHAO CHONG

Tongue which is contracted causing difficulty in speaking known as Yin rigidity: XIN SHU, SHAN ZHONG, HAI YUAN

Cracked and split lips which are bleeding and painful: CHENG JIANG, SHAO SHANG, GUAN CHONG (TH 1)

Scrofula which surrounds the neck as raised lumps and is known as Coiled Serpent Pestilence: TIAN JING (TH 10), FENG CHI, ZHOU QIAN (LI 12), QUE PEN (St 12), SHI XUAN

Chronic scrofula which extends to the chest and the axillary region known as Melon Vine Pestilence: JIAN JING, SHAN ZHONG, DA LING, ZHI GOU, YANG LING QUAN

Tumor at the root of the left ear known as Orchid Pouch Pestilence: YI FENG (TH 17), HOU XI, ZHOU QIAN

Tumor at the root of the right ear known as Honeycomb Pestilence: YI FENG, JIA CHE, HOU XI, HE GU

Redness, swelling, and pain at the root of the ear: HE GU, YI FENG, JIA CHE

Intractable redness and swelling of the neck and nape known as Nuchal Ulcer: FENG FU, JIAN JING, CHENG JIANG

Corneal opacity making it difficult to open the eye: JING MING (Bl 1), HE GU, GAN SHU, YU WEI (Extra point[27])

Wind rots the edges of the eye; when facing the wind it eleicits cold tears: ZAN ZHU, SI ZHU KUNG, ER JIAN (LI 2), XIAO QU KUNG

Swelling and pain due to Wind in the eye with protruding flesh involving the eyeball: HE LIAO (TH 22), JING MING, ZAN ZHU, GAN SHU, WEI ZHONG, HE GU, ZHOU QIAN, LIE QUE, ZHAO HAI, SHI XUAN

Swelling and pain in the teeth of both jaws: REN ZHONG, HE GU, LU XIN

Pain in the teeth of the upper jaw with inability to open the mouth: TAI YUAN, JIA CHE, HE GU, LU XIN (Ki 3)

Pain in the teeth of the lower jaw with pain, redness, and swelling in the cheek and neck: YANG XI, CHENG JIANG, JIA CHE, TAI XI

Deafness and a Qi lump which is sore and painful: TING HUI, SHEN SHU, ZU SAN LI, YI FENG

Tinnitus with itching or pain: HE GU, TING HUI, KE WANG REN (GB 3)

Splitting headache[28] with vertigo, protracted vomiting of Phlegm: BAI HUI, ZHONG WAN, TAI YUAN, FENG MEN

Kidney Deficiency headache where the head feels heavy and cannot be lifted: SHEN SHU, BAI HUI, TAI XI, LIE QUE

Vertigo due to Rebellious Phlegm with a sense of murkiness in the head and eyes: DA DUN, GAN SHU, BAI HUI

Pain in the head and neck known as Genuine Head Wind: SHANG XING (GV 23), BAI HUI, NAO KONG (GB 19), YONG QUAN, HE GU

Sudden redness, swelling, and pain in the eyes: ZAN ZHU, HE GU, YING XIANG (LI 20)

Yang's Symptomology:

Stroke with hand tremors: ZHONG ZHU, YANG CHI (TH 4), QU CHI, BA XIE

REN MAI

LIE QUE is situated bilaterally on the Lung Channel. It lies one CUN, five FEN above the inside of the wrist and when the hands are interlocked the finger rests ina hollow between the bones. It is needled to a depth of five FEN. LIE QUE controls disorders of the subcardiac region of the ribs and the Five ZHANG. ZHAO HAI is its corresponding point of influence.

Symptomology (according to Xi Jinag-yue): Hemorrhoids, malaria, swollen bowels and dysentery, hemoptysis, coughing up Phlegm, toothache, swollen throat, difficult urination, soreness of the Heart, chest, and abdomen, and choking. Futhermore, it treats postpartum aphonia, lumbar pain, acute hemorrhage and cold umbilicus, dead fetus hich won't descend, and Cold in the diaphragmatic region. LIE QUE dissolves carbuncles of the breast. In treating the following symptoms, first needle LIE QUE; then choose the other appropriate points (according to Xu).

Malodorous nasal discharge known as rhinorrhea: QU CHAI (Bl 4), SHANG XING, BAI HUI, FENG MEN, YING XIANG

Nasal polyps which obstruct the nasal airways: YIN TANG, YING XIANG, SHANG XING, FENG MEN

Injury by pathogenic Wind causing facial redness, fever, and headache: TONG LI, QU CHI, JUE GU, HE GU

Common cold due to injury by pathogenic Wind with a full cough: SHAN ZHONG, FENG MEN, HE GU, FENG FU

Injury by pathogenic Wind where there is fever in the four limbs and headache: JING QU (Lu 8), QU CHI, HE GU, WEI ZHONG

Intra-abdominal and intestinal pain with incessant diarrhea: NEI TING, SAN YIN JIAO

Red and white dysentery; the abdomen is cold and painful: SHUI DAO (St 28), QI HAI, WAI LING (St 26), TIAN SHU, SAN YIN JIAO, ZU SAN LI

Pain, swelling, and redness of the breasts and the front of the chest: SHAO ZE (SI 1), DA LING, SHAN ZHONG

Swollen, painful breast carbuncle due to suckling: ZHONG FU (Lu 1), SHAN ZHONG, SHAO ZE, DA DUN

Abdominal coldness with incessant diarrhea: TIAN SHU, ZHONG WAN, GUAN YUAN, SAN YIN JIAO

Dysmenorrhea and hemorrhage: GAN SHU, SHEN SHU, GE SHU, SAN YIN JIAO

Cold Phlegm cough with pain and obstruction in the chest and diaphragm: FEI SHU, SHAN ZHONG, ZU SAN LI

Intractable cough and coughing up bloody Phlegm: FENG MEN, TAI YUAN, SHAN ZHONG

Asthma and dyspnea; Phlegm flourishes and obstructs the breathing: FENG LONG, SHU FU (Ki 27), SHAN ZHONG, ZU SAN LI

Rumbling asthma with urgent pain in the chest and diaphragm: YU ZHONG (Ki 26), TIAN TU, FEI SHU, ZU SAN LI

Rumbling asthma with thoracic fullness where the Lungs are distended and one cannot lie down: SHU FU, FENG MEN, TAI YUAN, ZHONG FU, ZU SAN LI, SHAN ZHONG

Nasal obstruction resulting in anosmia: YING XIANG, SHANG XING, FENG MEN

Slight, thin, clear nasal discharge and incessant sneezing: SHEN TING (GV 24), FEI SHU, TAI YUAN, ZU SAN LI

Breakthrough bleeding and agalactia: SHAO ZE, DA LING, SHAN ZHONG, GUAN CHONG

Ulcerated nipple known as Jealous Breast: RU GEN, SHAO ZE, JIAN JING, SHAN ZHONG

Squeezing, obstructed pain in the chest: DA LING, NEI GUAN, SHAN ZHONG, ZU SAN LI

The five types of goiter; these five types of neck goiter are known as: Stone Goiter, since it is hard like a stone; Qi Goiter, since it is soft as silk; Blood Goiter, since there are fine, threadlike blood vessels in it; Tendonous Goiter, since there is no bone; and Flesh goiter, since its form is sacklike: FU TU (LI 18), TIAN TU, TIAN CHUANG (SI 16), QUE PEN, SHU FU, YING SHU (Lu 1), SHAN ZHONG, HE GU, SHI XUAN (bleed)

Sores on the inside of the mouth and halitosis: SHI XUAN, REN ZHONG, JIN JIN, YU YE, CHENG JIANG, HE GU

Strong fever in the Triple Heater with sores on the tongue: GUAN CHONG, WAI GUAN, REN ZHONG, YING XIANG, JIN JIN, YU YE

Halitosis: SHAO CHONG, TONG LI, REN ZHONG, SHI XUAN, JIN JIN, YU YE

Summer Heat with high fever, choleric vomiting, and diarrhea: WEI ZHONG, BAI LAO, ZHONG WAN, QU CHI, SHI XUAN, ZU SAN LI, HE GU

Heatstroke with spontaneous sweating and difficult urination: YIN QU, BAI LAO, ZHONG WAN, WEI ZHONG, QI HAI, YIN LING QUAN

Acute infantile convulsions with spasms of the hands and feet: YIN TANG, BAI HUI, REN ZHONG, ZHONG CHONG, DA DUN, TAI CHONG, HE GU

Chronic infantile Spleen Wind; the eyes look straight upwards and there are spasms of the hands and feet and spitting up of saliva: DA DUN, PI SHU, BAI HUI, SHANG XING, REN ZHONG

Diabetes. There are three distinct types of diabetes: Obstructive emaciation, Middle Emaciation, and Kidney Emaciation. The SU WEN states that "when the Stomach is Deficient, the food is in contention and thus hunger is not sufficiently satisfied. When the Kidney is Deficient, drinking one hundred glasses (of liquid) will not quench the thirst and sex is not pleasurable." Thus there are three kinds of diabetes. When the Earth is parched and there is thirst, transformation is not possible and disease results: REN ZHONG, GONG SUN, PI SHU, ZHONG WAN, GUAN CHONG, ZHAO HAI (treats thirst which drinking will not quench), TAI XI (treats lack of sexual desire), ZU SAN LI (treats unsatisfiable hunger)

Black Colic abdominal pain and headache, fever and chillophobia, stiffness and pain in the back and lumbar region and inability to sleep lying down: BAI LAO, QI LAO YIN (GB 11), SHI XUAN, TIAN FU (GV 16), WEI ZHONG

White Colic abdominal pain, vomiting, and diarrhea, coldness of the extremities, the nails of the fingers are black and there is an inability to sleep while lying down: DA LING BAI LAO, DA DUN, SHI XUAN

Black & White Colic headache and perspiration, thirst, diarrhea, chillophobia, coldness of the extremities, and inability to sleep lying down. This is known as colic from Intestinal Entanglement. There may be borborygmus or abdominal noises: WEI ZHONG, SHAN ZHONG, BAI HUI, DAN TIEN, DA DUN, QIAO YIN (GB 1), SHI XUAN

Dizziness due to Blood Stagnation: REN ZHONG

Distention and knottedness in the chest and diaphragm: YONG QUAN, SHAO SHANG, SHAN ZHONG, NEI GUAN

Soreness and pain in the umbilical region: SHAN ZHONG, DA DUN, ZHONG FU, SHAO ZE (SI 1), TAI YUAN, SAN YIN JIAO

Distress and discomfort in the Heart: YIN LING QUAN, NEI GUAN

Tinnitus (like cicada sounds): SHAO CHONG, TING HUI, ZHONG CHONG, SHANG YING (LI 9)

Tirbid nasal discharge: SHANG XING, NEI GUAN, LIE QUE, QU CHI, HE GU

Fever due to injury by Cold: QU CHAI (Bl 4), NEI GUAN, LIE QUE, JING QU (Lu 8), HE GU

YIN QIAO MAI

ZHAO HAI is situated bilaterally on the Kidney Channel. It is located in a sitting position with the soles of the feet touching, in a hollow beneath the medial malleolus, and it is needled to a depth of one CUN, two FEN. It governs diseases of the Organs and Bowels and LIE QUE is its corresponding point of influence.

Symptomology (according to Xi Jiang-yue): Obstructions of the throat, urinary tract disorders, Stagnant Qi pain of the Urinary Bladder and intestinal rumbling, "foot jaundice", and alcoholic indigestion in the periumbilical region; vomiting and diarrhea, gastric upset and constrained bowel movements, difficult labor, coma, and stagnant lumps; frequent melena due to pathogenic Wind Heat in the intestines , Stagnant Qi lumps in the diaphragmatic region. ZHAO HAI will certainly achieve a positive effect. When treating the following symptoms, first needle ZHAO HAI as the controller; then choose other appropriate points.

Cystitis causing difficult urination: YIN LING QUAN, SAN YIN JIAO, GUAN CHONG, HE GU

Pain and chill in the lower abdomen with frequent urination: QI HAI, GUAN YUAN, SHEN SHU, SAN YIN JIAO

The seven "hernias" of the Urinary Bladder and "Running Piglet" symptomology: DA DUN, DAN TIEN, SAN YIN JIAO, YONG QUAN, ZHANG MEN, DA LING

Kidney edema with swelling moving upwards: DA DUN, QU QUAN, RANG GU, SAN YIN JIAO, GUI LAI (St 29), PANG GUANG SHU (Bl 28), SHEN SHU (Bl 23, moxa seven times)

Tautness and stricture of the breast occuring when there is "rushing Heart" pain: DAI MAI (GB 26), YONG QUAN, TAI XI, DA DUN

Incessant hematuria and pain in the genitals: YIN GU, YONG QUAN, SAN YIN JIAO

Spermatorrhea with a thick white emission and frequent urination: GUAN YUAN, BAI HUAN SHU (Bl 30), TAI XI, SAN YIN JIAO

Spermatorrhea with dreams: ZHONG JI (CV 3), GAO HUANG SHU, XIN SHU, RANG GU, SHEN SHU

Difficult labor; the infant clings to her mother's Heart (and therefore is) unable to descend; retained placenta: JU QUE (CV 14), HE GU, SAN YIN JIAO, ZHI YIN (Bl 67 with moxa)

Constipation in women: SHEN MAI, YIN LING QUAN, SAN YIN JIAO, TAI XI

Postpartum abdominal pain with incessant discharge: SHUI FEN, GUAN YUAN, GAO HUANG SHU, SAN YIN JIAO

Tired Qi and Blood in women with Heat in the Five Hearts; the entire body is painful and there is vertigo: SHEN SHU, BAI HUI, GAO HUANG SHU, QU CHI, HE GU, JUE GU

Geriatric Deficiency with cramping of the hands and feet and inability to move them: CHENG SHAN, YANG LING QUAN, LIN QI, TAI CHONG, CHI ZE, HE GU

Cholera with vomiting and diarrhea and cramping of the hands and feet: JING QU (Bl 64), ZU SAN LI, CHENG SHAN, QU CHI, WAN GU, CHI ZE, YANG LING QUAN

Damp Cold "foot Qi" with fever and severe pain: TAI CHONG, WEI ZHONG, SAN YIN JIAO

Kidney Deficiency "foot Qi" with redness, swelling, and unrelenting fever: QI CHONG (St 30), TAI XI, GONG SUN, SAN YIN JIAO, WEI ZHONG

Dry "foot Qi" with pain and soreness in the kneecap extending down to the medial malleolus and the five toes: XI QUAN (GB 33), KUN LUN, JUE GU, WEI ZHONG, YANG LING QUAN, SAN YIN JIAO

Edema resulting in distention and fullness from head to foot: QI HAI, ZU SAN LI, QU CHI, HE GU, NEI TING, XING JIAN, SAN YIN JIAO

Thinness of the abdominal wall, parasitic abdominal distention, and intractable asthma: SHAN ZHONG, QI HAI, SHUI FEN, ZU SAN LI, XING JIAN, SAN YIN JIAO

Extreme distention of the subcardiac region such that it resembles a basin: ZHONG WAN, SHAN ZHONG, SHUI FEN, SAN YIN JIAO

Edema of the face, eyes, and extremities which will not subside: REN ZHONG, HE GU, ZU SAN LI

Feminine Deficiency and emaciation with red and white leukorrhea: BAI LAO, SHEN SHU, GUAN YUAN, SAN YIN JIAO

Chronic uterine chill with inability to conceive: ZHONG JI, SAN YIN JIAO, ZO GONG (Extra point)

Normal menstruation, however dizziness and lower abdominal pain: YANG JIAO (GB 35), NEI TING, HE GU

Irregular menstruation with lower abdominal pain and soreness in virgins: SHEN SHU, SAN YIN JIAO, GUAN YUAN

Postpartum difficulty or difficult parturition: HE GU, SAN YIN JIAO, DU YIN (Extra point: on the transverse crease on the underside of the second toe)

Yang's Symptomology:

Parasites in the Qi and Blood: XING JIAN, GUAN YUAN, SHUI FEN, GONG SUN, QI HAI, LIN QI

Heat in the Five Hearts : NEI GUAN, YONG QUAN, SHI XUAN, DA LING, HE GU, SI HUA ("four flowers", Bl 17, 19)

Qi attacks causing chest pain: TONG LI, DA LING

Palpitations: XIN SHU, NEI GUAN, SHEN MEN

Obstruction in the throat: SHAO SHANG, FENG CHI, ZHAO HAI

Prolapse due to Deficiency of Yang: XIN SHU, RANG GU, SHEN SHU, ZHONG JI, SAN YIN JIAO

As to the above eight techniques, first needle the point which controls the symptoms, i.e. the "controlling point", then according to the focus of the illness, choose the other points of influence.

In intractable illnesses, the HE Sea points are certainly indicated. One must stop needling once the Qi has been obtained as this enables above and below to be joined until there is no pain. Afterwards withdraw the needle. Moxa may be used. All this notwithstanding, protocols still depend on the individual case and one should not rely on the needle alone.

CONCLUSION

Modern texts on TCM acupuncture, such as ESSENTIALS OF CHINESE ACUPUNCTURE, ACUPUNCTURE: A COMPREHENSIVE TEXT, and THE MERIDIANS OF ACUPUNCTURE[29], illustrate the Extraordinary vessels with the same thin black lines used for delineating the courses of the twelve main "organ" meridians. This is misleading. According to Michael Broffman, a more accurate representation would be to liken the eight Extraordinary vessels to the Everglades. The Everglades are a "river" more than a hundred miles wide. Within this vaste drainage system there are distinct channels whose course can be traced and which are named. These distinct channels or rivers exist within the larger flow of the Everglades. Although the state of circulation within these rivers is, to some extent, distinct, it is obviously also dependent upon the total amount of water percolating through the Everglades.

It is in just this way that the eight Extraordinary vessels regulate the flow of energy within the twelve meridians. They are the background flow of energy in the broad areas of the body which they percolate through. This is what, I believe, Li Yan was refering to when he called these vessels "the common pool of the twelve regular channels".

The eight Extraordinary vessels primarily circulate YUAN QI. YUAN QI is likewise the energy which moves and catalyzes all the other pure substances and energies of the organism. In a sense, the YUAN QI and the Extraordinary vessels are one and the same. When referred to as the Extraordinary vessels, the route and direction of flow is being emphasized. When referred to as the YUAN QI, the function is being emphasized. However, the route and the function are only different perspectives on a single reality, just as there is no river without water.

The YUAN QI and the Extraordinary vessels arise in the Kidneys. Embryologically it is my opinion that the Extraordinary vessels represent the original lines of cleavage in the dividing zygote. The CHONG MO then is the central polar axis. The YIN WEI/YANG WEI MO, YIN QIAO/YANG QIAO MO, and the DU MO/REN MO represent the longitudinal lines of electromagnetic force. And the DAI MO is the equator. As an extension of this simile it seems reasonable to suppose that the eight Extraordinary vessels might be used in order to balance the posture of the entire body similar to Rolfing, and, in fact, certain Japanese practitioners[30] have developed their use along these lines.

In any case, it is my opinion that modern practitioners, recognizing both the simplification of modern TCM acupuncture and the "herbalization" of its practice, should investigate in greater depth the potential of these eight Extraodinary vessels. Although Li Shi-zhen cross-referenced certain of Zhang Zhung-jing's herbal formulae with the Extraordinary vessels[31], still, they are primarily an acupuncture theory. It is also my experience that the conscious employment of these vessels is, as the ancients suggested, a higher or advanced practice of acupuncture. That is not to say, however, that their use is indicated in all situations. The practitioner must still make an accurate Chinese energetic diagnosis, a process that I have found all too often many American practitioners of so-called Chinese medicine are incapable of. The use of the eight Extraordinary vessels is not a catch-all panacea. Diagnostic indications suggesting an aberration or imbalance in one or more of the Extraordinary vessels are given in Woolerton & McLean's ACUPUNCTURE ENERGY IN HEALTH & DISEASE and also in "The Eight Extra Meridians" by Giovanni Maciocia.[32] However, if in fact an imbalance exists at the level of the Extraordinary vessels, manipulation of the twelve regular meridians will only achieve temporary and symptomatic relief. Therefore, not only is this an advanced level of practice, but it is also an indispensible one as well.

ENDNOTES

1 Anon., Beijing College of Traditional Chinese Medicine, "Clinical Application of the Crossing Points of Eight Extra Channels", MEDECINE TRADITIONELLE CHINOISE ET ACUPUNCTURE, Quebec, Vol. 7 #3, Nov. 1984, p. 22

2 Hammer, Leon, "Extraordinary Acupuncture Meridians: Homeostatic Vessels", AMERICAN JOURNAL OF ACUPUNCTURE, Vol. 8 #2, April-June 1980, p. 123

3 "Clinical Application of the Crossing Points...", op. cit., p. 24

4 Woollerton, Henry & McLean, Colleen J., ACUPUNCTURE ENERGY IN HEALTH AND DISEASE, Thorsons Publishers Ltd., Wellingborough, UK, p. 65-6

5 "Clinical Application...". op. cit., p. 22

6 Ibid., p. 25

7 Ibid., p. 25

8 Ibid., p. 24

9 Ibid., p. 24

10 Lu Gwei-djen & Needham, Joseph, CELESTIAL LANCETS, Cambridge University Press, Cambridge, London, etc., 1980, p. 270

11 Varieties of symptoms due to an accumulation of pathogenic Heat or Cold with Fluids (either Phlegm or Blood) in the chest or abdomen

12 Xu Yen-bai

13 Various enumerations of the differentiations of Heart pain have existed throughout Chinese medical history. The point here is not that there are five specific types of Heart pain but that this prescription treats all types of Heart pain.

14 The emphasis is on the rushing up of Qi.

15 This appears to be a Stagnant Qi pattern.

16 FAN WEI: a gastric disorder causing nausea. The BULLETIN OF THE ORIENTAL HEALING ARTS INSTITUTE, Vol. 10 #6, Sept. 1985, p. 236, defines FAN WEI as stomach cancer, a symptom of which is "vomiting food that has entered the stomach and remained there a while."

17 The following are specific differentiations of malaria as a general category. Malaria here means an infectious disease clinically characterized by periodic attacks of chills, high fever, and sweating at regular intervals.

18 Literally "sprinkling fever"

19a BAI LAO: there are classical references to this point being either GV 14 or Bl 11. Given its use in this text, identifying it as GV 14 makes the most sense and it has been translated here as such.

19b Blood JIA: "masses in the hypogastrium and hypochondrium" according to CHINESE ENGLISH TERMINOLOGY OF TRADITIONAL CHINESE MEDICINE, Hunan Science & Technology Press, 1981, p. 570

20 Visceral toxicity causing melena: the symptom complex of the passage of dark blood clots with bowel movements accompanied by reduced appetite and lassitude caused by an accumulation of pathogenic Damp Heat in the Intestines

21 According to Huang Pao-chin, inflammation of both sides of the tonsils

22 Headwind: "persistent and recurrant headaches, refractory to treatment", CHINESE ENGLISH TERMINOLOGY, op. cit. , p. 539

23 In the middle of the transverse crease of the phalangeal joint of the little finger, dorsal aspect

24a Thundering headache: the patient experiences a thundering noise in the ears during headache, with redness, swelling, and pain of the head and face. It is usually caused by upward invasion of a Damp pathogen.

24b According to Huang Pao-chin, too much work or exercise may create an Internal Wind which may move throughout the body causing pain and discomfort in various locations.

25 Five Tigers: the interphalangeal joints of the index and ring fingers of both hands; moxa five times.

26 Located at the root of the tongue between JIN JIN and YU YE

27 Between the outer canthus and TONG ZI LIAO (GB 1)

28 Literally "like thunder"

29 Mann, Felix, THE MERIDIANS OF ACUPUNCTURE, William Heinemann Medical Books Ltd., London, 1972

30 Dr. Nagatomo

31 Zerox reprints of THE PULSE STUDIES OF THE LAKESIDE MASTER & HIS CLASSIC OF THE EXTRAORDINARY CHANNELS, Wen Guang Pictures & Books Ltd., place & date ?

32 Maciocia, Giovanni, "The Eight Extra Meridians, Parts One & Two" collected in an untitled and undated anthology of essays published by THE JOURNAL OF CHINESE MEDICINE, UK

JIN ZI-JIU'S MEDICAL CONTEMPLATIONS

Excerpts from the JIN ZI-JIU ZHUAN JI

Biographical and Bibliographical Introduction: The following excerpts have been translated from JIN ZI-JIU ZHUAN JI coedited by the Zhe Jiang Province Chinese Medical Research Institute and the Zhe Jiang Province Jia Xing District Health Office and published by the Peoples' Health Publishing Society in Beijing in 1982. This is a collection of Jin Zi-jiu's medical essays. Jin Zi-jiu lived from 1870 to 1921. He was born in Hangzhou and lived in eastern China his entire life. From his first years studying Chinese medicine and throughout his career, Dr. Jin worked assiduously at his profession. Not only was he well versed in all the ancient classics but he also applied himself wholeheartedly to diagnosing and treating difficult cases. It is also to his credit that he treated poor people as well as the rich and even contributed from his own pocket for the treatment of widows and orphans. As a doctor, scholar, and gentleman, Dr. Jin Zi-jiu is worthy of our attention and respect.

Dr. Jin's writings translated below are theoretical contemplations on various topics of classical Chinese medicine. According to Huang Pao-chin, Dr. Jin's essays are multilayered in meaning. The Chinese language lends itself to multimodal inference. Due to the inherent structural dissimilarity between Chinese and English, most of the subtle semantic inferences and allusions do not come through translation. Therefore it is possible that a classically-trained Chinese doctor reading Jin Zi-jiu might derive a different or deeper insight from these essays than the American reader reading these translations. However, even on the somewhat superficial level of this translation, there is much food for thought for American practitioners of Chinese medicine. These excerpts were translated by Micheal Helme and edited by Bob Flaws.

ROOTS AMONG THE FIVE ZANG

The Roots of the Five ZANG are the Spleen and the Kidneys, while the Branches and leaves are the Heart and the Lungs. When the Spleen is Insufficient it does not Transform the Pure Essence, but (rather) creates Turbid Phlegm.

When the Kidneys are Insufficient they do not Grasp the Righteous Qi (ZHEN QI) and dyspnea results. When the Lungs are Insufficient they do not smoothly Dispatch the Qi and the Qi Rebels in coughing. When the Heart is Insufficient the SHEN and the Will are not cared for and float adrift. The Kidneys are the mother of the Liver. The Lungs are the son of the Spleen. When the Kidneys are ill, the Liver loses its Moistening and Nurturing power. When the Spleen is sick, Lung Metal loses the mechanism which creates Qi. Wood stops Earth and Metal can control Wood. But when Deficient Metal is unable to Spread Wood, the strength of Wood's Qi must Level the rebellion. Otherwise Wood Insults Earth and Below there is diarrhea. If Metal is punished by Fire, Above experiences coughing and choking. When one knows how to grasp the Roots, the leaves and Branches cannot wither.

SPLEEN AND STOMACH, THE FOUNDATION OF POSTNATAL (QI)

As the Essence and Mind of man look to Earth as their abode, the ten thousand things look to Earth as their Root. When the Postnatal Stomach and Spleen attain force, the Righteous (ZHEN) and Original (YUAN) Qi are able to fulfill themselves. Man's Qi mechanism and Yin-Yang rest entirely upon the authority of the Stomach-Spleen. Man's Heavenly Righteous Qi is all in the Stomach. Therefore, Nurturing the Stomach's JIN-Fluid is the plain way to tonify Deficiency.

The Stomach rules holding the food. The Spleen governs Transportation and Transformation. The Stomach is Yang Earth, while the Spleen is Yin Earth. Stomach Yang relies on Spleen Yin for Moistening just as Spleen Yin borrows Stomach Yang for Warming. The Spleen and Stomach serve as Exterior and Interior and are the spring of Postnatal Creation and Transformation. By the one act of treating the Spleen, three good results will come. First, flourishing Spleen Qi is like a blue sky on a wonderful day with dragons and lightning subdued from attack. Secondly, flourishing Spleen Qi allows Essence and Qi to roam overflowingly and supply upwards to the Lungs. And finally, flourishing Spleen Qi allows the Pure Essence of Water and Grain to replenish the Blood before it reaches exhaustion.

The hundred diseases of the four seasons all originate in the Stomach. As the Stomach gets Grain, improvement comes. Therefore, if the diet is improved one inch, the disease pathogen is forced back one inch. Consequently, in chronic illnesses, sleep and diet must be emphasized. Sleeping unsettled and eating irregularly, how will the JIN YE (Fluids) regenerate, and what will maintain the mechanisms of production? After illness, readjust the Stomach and Spleen. Relying on the Middle Qi to gain authority, the dietetic pathogens and Excesses can transform and resolve themselves. Moreover, Liver Yang, Qi, and Fire will not be able to float upwards.

By Facilitating Ascension the Spleen is made healthy. By Facilitating Descension the Stomach is Harmonized. Li Dong-yuan emphasized Raising Yang Qi. His cure is in the Spleen. Zhang Zhong-jing emphasized Descending JIN Fluids. His cure is in the Stomach. It is good to arouse the Stomach. This services the Creation of JIN and the Nurturing of YE. It is also good to establish a healthy Spleen because the key is in Raising the Pure and Descending the Turbid.

EXPLANATION OF QI MECHANISM

The classics say: "Spleen Qi Disperses the Pure Essence which returns upwards to the Lungs." This is the ascension of Mother Earth's Qi. The Lungs rule the junctions and thereby the flow of Water in its descent to the Bladder. This is Heaven's Qi descending. Inhaling and exhaling are dominated by the Kidneys and the Lungs. The Lungs exhale Qi. The Kidneys inhale. While the Lungs Clear and Purify the Qi, ascending and descending occur unobstructed and breathing is natural. But when rebellion or chaos sets in, the natural state is turned around. More specifically, Rebellion means difficult respiration and Chaos is turbulent ascension and descension. When Clear Yang Qi cannot filter through, then the flows of rising and falling stagnate and the distribution of Fluids becomes erratic. Thus, the Clear that rises and the Turbid that descends rely entirely on the Middle WAN's motion. Because the Spleen and Stomach reside in the Middle, they are the real directors of inhaling and exhaling. With the Middle WAN wide open, the ascension and descension of Clear and Turbid cannot be impeded. The Bowels and Orifices flow freely. Thus the rise and fall of the Stomach and Spleen dictate the whole body's Qi mechanism. If the Middle Burner's foundation is not set in solid rock, then ascending and descending are shifty. Breathing is too stuffy and the Qi that is grasped does not collect in the Reservoirs. Thus the Refined Essence seeps out but is not Spread properly. Wrong steps are taken in all directions. The Yin and Yang rebel chaotically.

BODY TYPES

Plump, fat people with flaccid muscles and white skin are clearly Yang Deficient constitutionally. Thin, lanky people with poor complexion are beyond doubt Yin Deficient. People past adolescence with a frail constitution are lacking a tree-like foundation. In thin, timid types, the Yin is irrevocably Deficient and Fire will blaze due to this Deficiency. This scenario is quite common. A large, tall person is likely Yang Deficient. If such a person imbibes in tea and alcohol, they must have Internal Dampness. As Phlegm and Damp increase, the Yang must suffer because of it.

EXPLANATION OF YING, WEI, FEVER, AND CHILLS

When a new pathogen moves in from the outside while a latent pathogen moves out from the inside, both Interior and Exterior can be diseased and both Yin and WEI can be damaged. If YING is struggling, then there is Cold; while WEI struggling brings Heat. WEI is an aspect of Qi; YING an aspect of Yin. When Qi and Yin are Insufficient, YING and WEI are unsteady. Therefore, fever and chills switch back and forth. When Damp Wind Obstructs the meridians, the Flow of WEI Qi is impeded. YING and WEI tend to pool separately which again results in chills and fever.

The Spleen is the spring of the YING, just as the Stomach is (the spring) of the WEI. When the Stomach and Spleen are Empty and Deficient, YING and WEI have no reserves. Deficient YING then creates Heat and Deficient WEI creates Cold. YING and WEI are both forms of Qi. They circulate night and day without ceasing. So when both are Deficient, fever and chills do not stop at sunset.

With Phlegm and Excessive Fluid drifting in the meridians, they clog (their flow) and produce pain. When meridian Qi is obstructed, so is YING Qi. Therefore fever and chills come on like malaria. The muscles and meridians are all associated with YING and WEI. With flowing YING and WEI they are peaceful. But when the body runs hot and cold, it is because YING and WEI flood and recede.

Righteous Yin is plundered by Hot pathogens and due to this YING and WEI lose accordance. As YING gradually becomes Deficient, a fever will emerge. And as WEI becomes Deficient, chills ensue. Thus this is where chills and fever struggle and is not an indicator of the pathogen's status.

EXPLANATION OF WIND DAMAGE TO DEFICIENT LUNGS

When YING and WEI are dispersed and scanty they provide rickety fortifications. External Cold pathogens take advantage of this weakness to muster forces and entrench. Wind attacks the Upper. Therefore the nose portals either close up or are opened. Cold attacks the WEI. Therefore fever and chills ensue. As Clearing and Purifying Qi is increasingly injured, the Lungs lose their descending power. Thus coughing occurs but with little mucous. The Lungs command the YING and WEI and also lord over the whole body's Qi transformations. When the Lungs are Deficient, YING and WEI become incapable. So we can see why there are fever and chills. Furthermore, due to Deficient Lungs' (lack of) leadership, Qi Transformation stops responding to orders and this makes the limbs ache.

CONCERNS VIS A VIS SWEATING IN FEBRILE DAMP (DISEASES)

When the Qi of Heaven is hot and sticky there must be a big storm. When man's Qi is Hot and repressive there must be a big sweat. With no sweating how can a pathogen be resolved? One wants Heat's strength to be exposed and cooled. By servicing WEI's dispersing abilities, the Exterior will open and flow. Sweat will pour from the skin and pores and the strength of the Heat will start to withdraw. Thus Febrile Wind can be dispersed through the Exterior in one shot and damaging Cold can be cured with one plunge downwards. But Damp is a heavy, Turbid pathogen. Due to its Yin nature, Phlegm oozes downwards. Its basic nature is sticky; so everything gets smudged and it is not curable in one sweating.

Dampness injures Qi and transforms into Heat which then steams the YE Fluids and sweat flows. After the Exterior has perspired, subsequent diaphoresis may damage it. Excessive sweating should be avoided because Qi and YE Fluids will be injured. Then the JIN YE will not moisten anywhere and ascending and descending flows will be dammed up. In the spaces between top and bottom, inside and outside, Stagnant pathogens will fester uninhibited. Qi and YING will be completely cut off. All three Burners will be affected and ulcerations and swellings will emerge as both JIN and YE are damaged. Sweat is transformed from Yin YE. Therefore excessive sweating must damage the Yin making it difficult to maintain the Righteous Yin as well as for the JIN YE to support the Upper Burner. Sweat is the Fluid of the Heart; so excessive sweating will lead to Heart Deficiency. Since Yang lends agility to the SHEN, if Yang meets encumberment, the SHEN is hurt. Eventually the SHEN dims and the patient will crave lying down which means the Turbid Damp pathogen is deceptively obstructing Internally. When sweat pours like rain, the superficial Yang is dispersed or liberated to the outside. Thus it is said, for Febrile Damp, sweat lots, but think of creating waves of sweat. With profuse sweating, protect against fainting. If fainting occurs, protect against separation of Yin and Yang. For patients with Dampness, avoid sweating them too much. Otherwise spasm and convulsions will be caused. This is a famous rule from Zhang Zhong-jing.

EMPHASIZING FLUIDS IN WEN BING

The Six Pathogenic Evils all Transform into Fire. Fire is formless and spreads unbounded. It scorches upward and causes the Lungs to lose their Spreading and Purifying functions. Dryness is Transformed from Qi and Heat goes to the Stomach meridian. Therefore the Lungs and the Stomach must be the attacking ground for Febrile Wind. Dryness and Heat are expanding, flashy energies. Dryness damages the JIN and Heat injures the YE. The JIN is consumed by the Dry pathogen and the YE is fuel for a bright fire. The finite JIN YE is in a destitute situation then because the Heat is limitless and can rampage unbounded. Damage to the JIN YE is unavoidable in such a situation. Generally, after a Hot illness, one should promote Fluids. Heat symptoms are devastating to the Yin. As long as the Yin does not recover, the pathogen will not retreat.

One should push back the pathogen and Clear Heat by saving the Yin and creating the JIN. Because the JIN YE is fuel for Heat symptoms, Cooling and Moistening are the sure methods for treating Dry Heat. Immediately preserve Fluids with a prescription of Sweet and Cooling herbs. Moment by moment emphasize Fluids because, as they revive one inch, the Heat pathogens will recede one inch. As Fluids recover, Heat clears. The Yin aspect gradually improves day by day. Therefore Yang is self-contained and Heat will disperse of its own accord. Consequently, other than securing housing for the JIN and saving the YE, there is no other way to treat this problem. Otherwise, Yin stretches out more and more and is expended. Yang will then dominate and blaze. Qi, JIN, Yin, and YE are killed off. Yin is exhausted on the Interior as Yang continually moves out. The inside is parched dry and the Exterior departs, until finally Yin and Yang come apart.

DISCUSSION OF THE ORIGINS OF TB

The Lungs are like empty space. Called the Yellow Bell, their residence is like Heaven because its position is the highest. They are also the key to respiration and provide the doors and windows for sound. Among the ZANG FU, the Lungs hold court to Clear Qi, govern respiration, and lord over the entire body's Qi transformation. By nature they rule Descension. The Lungs are called the "tender" organ because they cannot withstand attacks from (External) pathogens. When (such) a pathogen triumphs, then everything rebels and becomes chaotic. The Lungs are (categorized) under Metal and amongst the Five Elements Fire can control Metal. As flames from Wood Fire leap higher, Metal Qi is increasingly injured and becomes Deficient. When too much Qi ascends, the descending function loses power, local pressure builds, and more Fire is created.

Qi and Fire originate together. If Qi rises, then Fire rises. If Qi rebels, then the Lungs rebel. Excess Fire leads to a dry cough. Thus the symptoms of coughing and laryngitis prove that Fire is unchecked. If Fire roars, then Phlegm will form and abundant Phlegm makes the Qi rebel. Fire is divided into Yin and Yang types, while Phlegm is differentiated into Excess and Deficiency. In chronic productive cough, Yin is run down and Fire arises from within Yin. For a chronic cough with much Phlegm, Phlegm must arise from Deficiency of the Middle. As far as Phlegm's pathological effect, it can change one hundred different ways, thus the old saying that one hundred diseases arise from Phlegm. Without Phlegm, Qi is not coughed up and with no coughing, the Qi is not rebellious. Qi and Phlegm mutually collide and migrate. Coughing with Qi ascending comes from substansive Phlegm obstructing the formless Qi.

Phlegm transforms from the Five Grains. Its origin is solely the Spleen. Coughing is produced by the Lungs but both Phlegm and coughing are due to rebellious Qi. As the Liver rises in Excess, the Lungs' capacity to descend is interfered with. Wood Fire damages Metal. Then Blood in the passageways follows in gurgling up and this is the sprouting of the signs of tubercular injury. As the body breathes, the Lungs' exhaling and the Kidneys' inhaling are both entirely dependent on the Lungs and Kidneys (mutually) irrigating each other. If there is the power to receive the Qi, then inhalation is rooted and exhalation grows as healthy fruit. If Kidney Water is Deficient, Liver Wood is not irrigated. The dragon Fire of the Kidneys flares upwards as the corresponding Fire in the Liver blazes. This Fire scorches upward. Therefore the Lungs are increasingly distended. Water below suffers and therefore the Kidneys are increasingly unable to grasp Qi. This then forms the circumstances for Lung damage.

THE TREATMENT OF DEFICIENCY DAMAGE HEMOPTYSIS

On the left, too much ascension; on the right, not enough descension. Therefore Wood's irrigation by Water is lost. Fire loses its restraint from Water. Then Wood and Fire (both) damage Metal. The Blood in the LUO is not tranquil. The Lungs and the LUO are damaged. As a result, Qi rebels and there is Blood in the Phlegm. Or, the Exterior is Cold and the Interior is Hot. Or, the eyes swell and sweat overflows. There is Phlegm coughing with a raspy voice. The throat and pharynx are painful due to obstruction (BI). The LUO pathways become obstructed and the Qi mechanism becomes blocked.

Qi and Blood mutually maintain and build up each other. If the Qi gets no Blood, then it disperses and is not unified. If the Blood gets no Qi, then it congeals and will not flow. Therefore Yin Qi moves as does Yin Fire. If Yin Fire spreads upward, then Yin Blood does also. Under these circumstances Qi and Blood seethe. Blood is expectorated due to lack of restraint because the Qi leads the Blood. So when Qi ascends, Blood overflows.

In treatment one should Infiltrate the Yang and Pacify the Yin in combination with restraining the Wood to Settle Metal, Clear the Dryness of Qi, Control the YING Qi's Fire, Clear the Qi and Settle the LUO, and Cool the Blood and stop bleeding. Or else, one can Promote the Grasping of Qi to help Blood absorption while getting rid of Stagnations to Create the New. If summer leads Damp Summer Heat to smoke and seethe, then Clear Summer Heat and Restrain Fire. If in addition there are runny stools not of the Excess variety and the patient has an exhausted, damaged countenance, then promote Earth to create Metal. The value of these treatment principles is their adaptability to individual cases.

DIFFERENTIATING EXCESS & DEFICIENCY APHONIA

Excess and Deficiency are (two) different kinds of muteness. Damaged JIN YE with Deficient Fire Blazing upwards causes Deficiency aphonia. Phlegm and Turbidity Flourishing on the Interior with Qi and Fire kicking upwards causes Excess aphonia. Sudden loss of voice is seldom due to Deficiency and is (most) commonly Excess (in nature). Because the Lungs rule the Light and Clear and heavy, Turbid Phlegm fouls the Lungs' capacity to clear and makes them Deficient, this also causes the sound to lose its hum. This is know as Excess Metal Not Ringing. Also, because the Liver meridian circulates the pharynx and the Kidney meridian circulates the larynx, when Kidney Liver Yin is Deficient the dragon spouts Fire and scorches the throat. The Kidneys are the child of the Lungs and a Deficient child drains its mother. Therefore Fire floats freely and strikes upwards at the Lungs. Lung Metal gets scorched, the Yellow Bell loses its resonance, and the sound loses its clarity because broken metal does not ring.

ESSENTIALS (FOR UNDERSTANDING) PHLEGM & STAGNATION OF FOOD & WATER

TAN Phlegm (discolored Phlegm) and YIN Phlegm (clear Phlegm) are (two) different categories but are basically of similar nature. When one looks at the source of TAN and YIN, it is Kidney Spleen Yang Deficiency for both. The Spleen does not provide transportation for the Stomach to move JIN YE Fluids and the Kidneys stop running the Stomach's sluicegate. Therefore the Dampness from Water and Grain congest the Middle Burner. From local Yang Excess TAN is formed. From Yin, YIN is formed. Straining the Spleen and sitting in the Lungs, this is where cough and asthma come from.

YIN Phlegm is divided into Internal and External types. Spleen Deficiency creates External YIN. Kidney Deficiency creates Internal YIN. Therefore Internal YIN is under the Kidneys and External YIN is under the Spleen.

TAN and YIN overstuff the Qi mechanism. Since ascension and descension lose their regularity, sometimes too much Qi rises bringing on asthma. (Other times) too much (Qi) descends bringing on edema. Qi and TAN circulate and collide with each other. When Qi circulates, so does TAN. When Qi moves, the rebellion emerges as cough. When Qi ascends, the TAN is expectorated. When the Lungs and the Stomach both tend to ascend, YIN and TAN become (even) harder to hold down. (These pathogens rarely descend.) Therefore problems in the Qi mechanism most likely manifest upwards.

The Lungs govern exiting Qi. The Kidneys govern grasping Qi. Therefore, Qi rebelling up with no asthmatic signs is not due to the Kidneys. Ascending Qi creating coughing is due to the Lungs. In Deficient Kidneys Unable to Grasp the Qi, Qi does not return to the well. The asthma is severe and there is difficulty lying down.

As for TAN, it is (also) divided into Excess and Deficiency. Wind Damp obstructing the Qi ferments into TAN or Excess TAN. Kidney Water striking rebelliously (on the other hand) ferments into Deficiency TAN. If the TAN is not salty flavored, it is not due to Water gurgling up. If it is foul and green, then there is Heat in the Lungs as well as in the Stomach. If the TAN stinks, it is from YIN Phlegm rotting above the diaphragm and transforming into Heat. Foamy, thick TAN in the early morning changing to runny TAN is Damp Spleen and Stomach TAN. If there is a rattling sound in the throat that is not easily expectorated, quite pasty and rubbery, then this is not Deficiency TAN.

KE and SUO (are commonly combined to mean cough but) are (actually) two technical terms with distinct definitions. KE comes from the Lungs and is due to Dryness in the Upper Burner. SUO comes from the Spleen and is due to Dampness in the Middle. Cough without TAN is KE; whereas, a phlegmatic cough is SUO.

The Spleen is the fountain of Phlegm. The Lungs are the vessel that holds the Phlegm. We can see that the Lungs are the Branch and the Spleen is the Root. The Kidneys rule the grasping of the Qi. In acute asthma, the Lungs are the flow but the Kidneys are the originating spring.

YIN Phlegm is Yin-natured so it tends to settle. Substansive YIN sticks to the Middle. Without Bitter and Fragrant herbs how can it be separated? Without Sweet and Warm herbs how can it be dried? Benefitting the Qi and Warming Yang are the bases for treating TAN.

A healthy Spleen and Stomach Ascend the Pure and Descend the Impure. When ascension and descension are well adjusted, how can Dampness clog the works? With the Stomach and Spleen raising and lowering the Qi properly the Qi will not stagnate nor will TAN form.

Extra Qi leads to Fire, but by restraining Fire the Qi remains calm. TAN follows Qi when it rises but is still as (long as) Qi is peaceful, which thus allows it to sink. Because cough (KE) comes from Qi, calming the Qi settles the Tender Organ. In treating KE cough, one only has to calm the Qi. Then the KE cough will take care of itself. Calming the Qi (also) helps TAN to move on its way. Calming exhaled Qi in the Upper Burner allows the YIN and TAN to transform themselves. Grasping inhaled Qi in the Lower Burner allows asthma and panting to level themselves.

A SHALLOW DISCUSSION OF STOMACH DISEASE

The Middle WAN is like Mother Earth. The Stomach resides in the Middle. It governs treasuring and grasping and commands the Six Bowels. When the Stomach Qi is regulated, food is accepted abundantly and the Qi mechanism is healthy. (Then) nothing can undermine the Middle. If Heat enters the Stomach, then Stomach Fire flash bakes the Qi. The WAN rumble and easily hunger. Like an unextinguishable fire, the more one eats, the more the fire roars (borborygmus). When the Stomach is Cold, the flow of Qi is impeded, ascending and descending become clogged, Upper and Lower lose communication, the Middle WAN develops lumpy obstructions, Clear Yang is stopped up, Turbid Yin congeals, the Middle JIAO is fettered, the Stomach WAN becomes painful, and Water starts spreading. The WAN is full and stuffy. Burping signifies the Qi is spreading unevenly. Chronic pain enters the LUO and follows them into the intercostal spaces. Next the pain moves to the shoulders or else there is vomiting and no defecation. The digestion may become unaccomodating or there may be (abdominal) distention. This is know as Nine Orifices Unharmonious and is mostly a Stomach illness.

When the Stomach is yielding, it is regulated. When the Bowels are open, they are usable. With regulated Stomach Qi, rising Yang does not explode upwards. When the Bowel Qi communicates, pathogenic Heat does not stay in the Stomach. In measures for Opening the Bowels, the main thing is Promoting Lubrication because, with Qi mechanism working and orifices open, condensations from the Upper Burner's mist can also move downwards. Thus, diseases of the ZANG Organs are related to treasuring and diseases of the FU Bowels are related to openness. If the Stomach's route for descension is not clear, then its drainage through the Intestines loses proper measure. Therefore ascension and descension stagnate and coagulate. Thus the hundred diseases of the four seasons begin with the Stomach and the whole case for treating pain by opening is as simple as Dredging and Transporting.

ON TREATING DIARRHEA

The Spleen governs healthy transportation. The Stomach governs healthy reception. The Spleen should rule ascension when healthy, just as the Stomach should rule descension. Li Dong-yuan emphasized Raising Yang Qi and he accomplished this through the Spleen. When the Spleen and Stomach have healthy transportation, Water and Grain are plentiful and beauteous. There is a basis for growth. But if the Qi of the Middle loses its transportation, this foundational pillar crumbles. Then Deficiency and Excess enmesh and rising and falling rebel into chaos. When little of Clear Yang ascends, the bowel movements are either unformed or runny. When little of Turbid Yin descends, the abdomen will have either lumps or distention. As ascension and descension of the Middle Burner become increasingly stagnant, it slimes into the Lower Burner and creates stagnation. The Stomach and Spleen lose harmony. The Qi mechanism is stopped up. The WAN is full and the abdomen aches. Less transportation occurs. The Clear and Turbid are not separated and eventually diarrhea ensues.

The Stomach is Yang Earth just as the Spleen is Yin Earth. Stomach Yang depends on the Spleen Yin for moistening in the same way that Spleen Yin depends on Stomach Yang for warming. This is the Stomach-Spleen's Exterior-Interior relationship and the source of Postnatal Creation and Transformation. Treatment involves encouraging and cheering the Middle Burner, helping the Spleen and Stomach, reviving the Clear and draining the Turbid, and Regulating ascension and descension. If the Intestines and the Stomach have Stagnations, they should be Opened and Cleared since the FU Bowels are happy when open. If the Stomach and Spleen are Deficient, they should be Tonified and Cleared because ZANG Organs should not let their prized contents dribble away. When the Qi has already prolapsed, if the Qi starts flowing again, will not the problem just get worse? With Yin on the decline, if one moves out Stagnations, will not the JIN YE become exhausted? Thus, if Stomach Yin is damaged, Stomach Fluids have been hurt and the Middle Yang is in decline. In order to aid Stomach Qi, Promote Fire to Create Earth. Then the Creation of Postnatal Qi will flourish and the Grasping of Grain will become more efficient. Therefore the JIN YE can brim and grow and Qi and YING will gradually become full.

ON TREATING DYSENTERY

Dysentery is of two kinds: Deficiency and Excess. If diarrhea precedes the dysentery, then a Spleen illness has moved to the Kidneys. If one comes down with (dysentery) in the Fall or Summer, the initial illness is probably Excess and Damp. After a chronic illness, the dysentery is probably Cold and Deficient. A protracted Spleen illness will eventually damage the Kidneys. The appendix does not separate the Pure and the Turbid. The Pure can not ascend but the Deficient Qi prolapses. This leads to damaged Blood and the dysentery will be red (i.e. contain blood). The Large Intestine no longer acts as a sluicegate and the dysentery is immeasurably painful. Food is poorly assimilated and the Interior is tense and later heavy. The Spleen and the Kidneys are mother and origin of the ten thousand things. These two organs are the important foundation (of life). If diarrhea prevails, then the Spleen will be damaged and if the dysentery prevails, then the Kidneys will be damaged. When the Spleen and Kidneys are damaged, the foundation is very shaky. When the MING MEN has no cooking power and Mother Earth's transportation is unhealthy, where is the basis for creating and disseminating energy? How will the diarrhea and dysentery stop?

Fire is the mother of Earth. For a Deficient son, tonify the mother. Promoting Fire strengthens movement. Tonifying Earth improves the power of absorption. Building Fire to Create Earth is necessary since by making Fire strong this allows transportation to go unchecked and ascension and descension occur spontaneously. This solidly Benefits the Qi and reliably stops the diarrhea and dysentery.

ON TREATING JAUNDICE

When Damp and Heat become yellow, Qi stagnates and does not project. Due to Damp's sticky nature, the Spleen is constricted and the Stomach is blocked. If constricted for long with no change, then everything changes into Phlegm. Phlegm (then) flows into the LUO and the Qi gets stopped. By being stopped up, the Qi causes pain. The pain is obviously Tai Yin Spleen meridian pain (because it is usually right-sided, subcostal pain) and since the Liver meridian disseminates through the intercostal spaces, as pain extends to there the Liver meridian is involved also. Because the Middle Burner holds on to the Dampness, the Clear Yang cannot expand. Thus very little of the Pure rises and this jams ascension and descension. When Jue Yin Qi is abundant, Stomach Earth gets hurt. Transportation loses harmony and Grain assimilation is restricted. Spleen Yang is crowded together and loses its edge. The Pure Essences from Water and Grain are easily scorched and turn to Dampness which becomes yellow. Interior and Exterior lose harmony. This is why fever and chills occur. Qi and Blood lose their patency and sometimes there is space in the abdomen and sometimes it is distended and painful.

Basic treatment principles are to Clear the Heat and Rid Dampness, Regulate the relation between the Liver and Spleen, Service the Qi's patency *vis a vis* the Spleen's transportation function. If this is done, the Damp pathogen will not attack but will self-destruct. Wood and Earth will be harmonious and (even) without treatment, YING and WEI will attain accord.

A DISCUSSION OF EDEMA

Why is edema classified (as a symptom of) Lung and Spleen (imbalance)? Because the Foot Tai Yin Spleen elevates Water and Grain while the Hand Tai Yin Lungs regulate the downward flow of Water. When the movement and channeling of Water occur spontaneously the sea flows but makes no waves. If either the Spleen or the Lung Qi is not active, then Water gets locked in the Stomach. Interior and Exterior are flooded and no place escapes the deluge. But are we to believe that this is all due to the Lungs and the Spleen?

Another important factor is the Kidneys because the Kidneys are the floodgate of the Stomach. The Stomach is the Sea of Grain and Water. Therefore all Water diseases must have some root in the Stomach. The Kidneys govern Opening and Closing. When Kidney Qi has sufficient Yang the floodgate opens. But with Excess Yang the gates crash open and Water runs straight down and out. When Yin is sufficient the gates come together, but when Excess they tightly shut up. Water congeals and edema forms. The classics say: "The Kidneys (are) the Root; the Lungs (are) the Branch." In other words, edema comes from the Lungs, Spleen, and Kidneys. Helping Kidney Qi Recieve and Grasp keeps Water from sloshing over. The Kidneys and the Bladder are Interior-Exteriorly related. Therefore, if the Bladder flourishes, then Qi transformation self-regulates and the Water canals are maintained on their own.

THREE METHODS FOR TREATING QI

There are three sources for treating the Qi. One method is Clearing the Lungs. With clear Lungs the whole body's Qi spreads and settles down. Another is to Clear the Stomach. A clear Stomach allows Chest Qi to descend. The third is to Clear the Bladder. When Bladder Qi is pure, inhaled Qi can be grasped by the Kidneys. When the Qi is Clear and the Source is Pure, all transportation and movement take place naturally and one is blessed with the power of peace.

A LIGHT DISCUSSION OF TREATING WIND BY FIRST NOURISHING BLOOD

Blood is a shaped substance that floods the hundred arteries, makes tendons supple, and allows the limbs to move. When the Blood is Deficient, the twelve meridians lose their nourishment. Being unable to nourish the JING and LUO, the arteries wither. (This) results in either pain or BI. Blood Not Nourishing Tendons makes the joints and knuckles sore. When the substansive Blood is injured, formless Qi is obstructed. Because the Qi does not fill the meridians they become blocked. And because the Blood does not nourish the tendons, the Blood stagnates. As the JING LUO fail to maintain their shape, Wind and Dampness superimpose on the Deficient situation and cause BI. Wind pathogen is the disease's Branch, either paralysing the limbs or making the joints sore. So it is said, "To cure Wind, first Nourish the Blood. When the Blood marches, the Wind retreats in defeat."

AN ANALYSIS OF TINNITUS

The classics say: "The Kidneys open in the ear." If the Kidneys are Deficient, then tinnitus occurs. So the theory goes. But this does not recognize that the Heart, Liver, and Gallbladder have LUO meridians around the ear. Rising Heart

Yang and Fire Collecting in the Gallbladder also produce tinnitus. Due to Kidney Water Not Irrigating Wood, Wood Fire blazes up and crackles in the orifice. Or, due to Liver Yang there is Internal Wind Drafting the Palace of Hearing. These are all possible analyses.

DISCUSSION OF THE EFFECTS OF ALCOHOL & TOBACCO

Tobacco has a Dry, Bitter energy which most easily damages Qi and attacks the Lungs. When the Lungs are injured, Qi loses its clearing and spreading (abilities) and the Yellow Bell loses resonance. Eventually it produces a cathartic cough or no tone whatsoever. Alcohol has a volatile nature that damages the SHEN and injure the Blood. Its energy is Hot and it leads to waste and decline. Alcohol first enters the Gallbladder-Liver where Gallbladder Fire explodes. The Qi loses its restraint and descension. Liver Yin is looted. The Blood becomes unsettled and as a result, rebellious ascension with vomiting of blood can occur. Moreover, alcohol is Damp as well as Hot. Dampness injures the Spleen. This creates Stagnant Food and Phlegm which easily gum the works. Heat damages the Lungs which easily causes coughing and asthma. If chronically Deficient with no recovery, Lung damage eventually effects the Kidneys. The Kidneys are a Water organ and once Kidney Water is Deficient, the Five Ministerial Fires increase many fold, wiping out Qi and YING. In short, smoking damages the Qi and drinking injures the Blood.

WANG LE-TING ON ACUPUNCTURE

Excerpts from JIN ZHEN WANG LE-TING

Biographical and Bibliographical Introduction: Dr. Wang Le-ting was born in 1894 and was still alive in 1983. He began practicing medicine in 1929 and in his more than fifty years of experience he has treated innumerable patients. Wang Le-ting has strictly adhered to the theories of Traditional Chinese Medicine and based on these theories he has created and developed many treatment methods and protocols. GOLDEN NEEDLE WANG LE-TING was published in Beijing in 1984. This book is a record of Wang Le-ting's special methods and insights into the practice of acupuncture. It was anonymously compiled by the Beijing Chinese Medical Hospital. The following are exerpts from GOLDEN NEEDLE WANG LE-TING chosen for translation for American practitioners of Oriental medicine because of their clinical usefulness and their historical significance. Wang Le-ting's style of treatment is a very clear example of consciously "herbalized" acupuncture. However, Dr. Wang also pays a great deal of attention to hand technique, the careful descrimination of tonification and dispersal, the location of points, and other such specifically acupuncture fine points. These exerpts have been translated by Michael Helme and edited by Bob Flaws.

OLD TEN NEEDLES

Stomach and intestinal diseases are commonly seen in clinical practice. For example, stomachache, abdominal pain, Stagnant Food, diarrhea, rocky stools, and other such symptoms are all problems which acupuncture and moxabustion treat effectively. After many decades of experience treating stomach and intestinal problems, Dr. Wang Le-ting has created an effective protocol called "Old Ten Needles" which carries into practice the dictum, "To treat the Root, first treat the Stomach". Old Ten Needles can also be used in other treatment plans as well.

The word old in the name Old Ten Needles has the following implications. First, it carries a sense of maturity and certainty. Secondly, because foods that Nourish the Stomach and Tonify the Spleen are all ripe (i.e. "old"), the word old is used here as an allusion to this concept. Moreover, the points used in the prescription are all traditionally important ones, in a sense "old" points. For these reasons we can see that the name Old Ten Needles is simple yet deep.

The points which make up this prescription are: SHANG WAN (CV 13), ZHONG WAN (CV 12), XIA WAN (CV 10), QI HAI (CV 6), TIAN SHU (St 25), NEI GUAN (Per 6), and ZU SAN LI (St 36). Since the last three points are needled bilaterally, ten points are needled altogether.

Dr. Wang has taken his theory on the treatment of digestive problems from Li Dong-yuan's PI WEI LUN (TREATISE ON STOMACH & SPLEEN) but uses acupuncture as his treatment modality.[1] His conceptual basis for structuring his Old Ten Needles treatment is founded on the herbal prescriptions DIAO ZHONG YI QI TANG (Decoction for Adjusting the Middle and Benefitting the Qi) and BU ZHONG YI QI TANG (Decoction for Tonifying the Middle and Benefitting the Qi), both from the PI WEI LUN. Of these, the concept of DIAO ZHONG YI QI TANG is relied upon more heavily. The ingredients of this formula are Astragalus, Ginseng, Licorice, Atractylodes, Bupleurum, Tangerine Peel, Cimicifuga, and Saussurea. This formula Benefits the Qi and Ascends the Yang while Strengthening the Spleen and Adjusting the Middle. It is also very effective for Adjusting and Promoting the Stomach and Intestines. Dr. Wang has based his point selection on this formula. Old Ten Needles is, therefore, indicated for Adjusting the Middle and Strengthening the Spleen, Promoting the Qi and Harmonizing the Blood, Ascending the Pure and Descending the Turbid, and Adjusting and Promoting the Stomach and Intestines.

Old Ten Needles relies on ZU SAN LI and ZHONG WAN as its primary points while the other points are prescribed as needed. ZHONG WAN sits in the middle of the Stomach and the other FU bowels. It is the meeting point of the Hand Tai Yang and Shao Yang, Foot Yang Ming, and the Ren Mai. It is also the meeting place of the Six FU and the MU point of the Stomach. When we say "meeting", it means a place where JING QI (Essence) collects. Therefore this point can open four channels. ZHONG WAN is also the place where the Foot Yang Ming Stomach channel Qi collects and it is indicated to Digest and Transform Water and Grain, Warm and Open FU QI, Ascend the Pure and Descend the Turbid, and Adjust and Promote the Middle Island's Qi mechanism (QI HUA).

ZU SAN LI is the HE sea point of the Foot Yang Ming. The term HE Sea point means that the channel Qi at this place is collected like a sea. The Foot Yang Ming is considered to have lots of both Qi and Blood and since SAN LI is the HE Sea point its use is rather broad, especially for diseases affecting the Six FU. Thus, tonifying SAN LI will Strengthen the Spleen and Harmonize the Stomach, Benefit the Qi, and Ascend the Pure. Dispersal at SAN LI is good for Lowering Rebellion and Transforming the Turbid, as well as Opening and Adjusting the Intestines and FU. Because the Stomach and Spleen are the Root of Postnatal (Qi), Dr. Wang has often said, "For the one hundred diseases, don't forget ZU SAN LI."

ZHONG WAN and ZU SAN LI in combination have the following indications: they Adjust the Middle and Benefit the Qi, Ascend the Pure and Descend the

the Turbid, and Adjust and Promote the Stomach and Intestines as well as the Qi and Blood. The other points (in the Old Ten Needles prescription) are discretionary and can be added to complement and strengthen the effects of these two main points.

SHANG WAN, ZHONG WAN, and XIA WAN are commonly called the Three WAN. SHANG WAN is located at the upper mouth of the Stomach, is under the Stomach's Connecting LUO to the Spleen, and is the meeting place of the Foot Yang Ming, Hand Tai Yang, and Ren Mai. It can open the door of the Stomach and FU to aid the reception and grasping of food and drink allowing them to enter the Stomach. XIA WAN is at the lower mouth of the Stomach and is the meeting point of the Foot Tai Yang and Ren Mai. It can Warm and Open the Stomach and Intestines, Benefit the Qi, and Descend Rebellion. Used together, the Three WAN Adjust and Promote Stomach and FU for Grasping, Ripening, and Receiving Water and Grain. Because of this, Dr. Wang emphasizes treating the Stomach and Spleen.

QI HAI is also called DAN TIEN or DAN ZAO. Because of its name we can see it is a Sea of Qi. By creating and issuing YUAN QI and Steaming and Moving QI HUA[2], it helps the transportation and transformation mechanism. It is also able to Open and Adjust the Ren Mai as well as Warm and Solidify the Lower Source Qi. When used in conjunction with ZHONG WAN, it helps to Benefit the Qi and Ascend Yang.

TIAN SHU is a point on the Foot Yang Ming channel. It is the MU point of the Large Intestine and the street for Qi in the abdomen. By "street" it is implied that Qi and Blood commonly traverse this broad expanse. Its effect is to Separate the Dregs from Water and Grain, Eliminate and Drain the Accumulations and Stagnations, and Adjust and Benefit the Spleen Qi. When used with ZHONG WAN, it is able to Adjust the Stomach and Intestines and Improve Transportation and Transformation. When used with QI HAI, it can help settle the Lower Burner Yang Qi and help the Stomach and Intestines ripen Grain and Water.

NEI GUAN is the Luo point of the Pericardium meridian. It goes to the Triple Heater. It Adjusts and Promotes the Triple Heater Qi mechanism, Settles the Mind, Harmonizes the Stomach, Expands the Chest, and Promotes Qi. Combined with ZHONG WAN and SAN LI, it can help Ascend the Pure and Descend the Turbid as well as Adjust and Promote the Qi mechanism.

OLD TEN NEEDLES' INDICATIONS & TRANSFORMATIONS

The parameters for employing Old Ten Needles are very broad. Its most important use is in the treatment of Stomach and intestinal disorders, while it has selective use in other illnesses. In sum, Old Ten Needles can be used for any Stomach and intestinal problem, whether Hot or Cold, Excess or Deficiency. When using Old Ten Needles, all one has to do is correctly apply the statement, "In Excess, disperse; in Deficiency, tonify." Examples are stomachache, abdominal pain, vomiting, diarrhea, Stagnant Food, constipation, and even prolapsed Stomach. From the point of view of clinical experience, we see that this includes the following western medical diseases: gastritis, stomach spasm, ulcers, enteritis, dysentery, parasitosis, indigestion, etc.

When used for Stomach pain, one treats Excess Cold or Excess Heat with dispersal technique. Whereas, for Deficiency Cold moxabustion is used. ZHONG WAN is most important here and it should be needled from one half to two CUN in depth. Dr. Wang needles ZHONG WAN relatively deeply. ZU SAN LI should be needled to a depth of two CUN. For Stomach Excess symptoms related to Qi, Blood, Phlegm, Coagulations, Food, Damp, or parasites, all require dispersal technique as well. For pain in the abdomen or diarrhea, TIAN SHU is the primary point and it should be needled to a depth of from one and a half to two CUN. For pain in the pelvis or gynecological diseases, QI HAI is the main point and should also be needled to a depth of from one and a half to two CUN. For Excess FU bowels and rocky constipation, TIAN SHU is again the main point. For ptosis of the Stomach, in addition to the standard Old Ten Needles, TIAN SHU should be needled through-and-through to ZHONG WAN. This raises the Stomach and FU. TIAN SHU can also be needled through to XIA WAN to push up the Stomach and FU. SHANG WAN and XIA WAN are usually needled to a depth of one and a half CUN.

Because the Spleen is the Postnatal Root and the Stomach is the Sea of Grain and Source of Creation and Transformation, adjusting the Stomach and Intestines influences the Qi and Blood systemically. As a result, illness in the Qi and Blood produces symptoms of Qi Deficiency and Blood Stagnation. By means of Adjusting and Promoting the Spleen and Stomach, there is a well-spring of Postnatal creation and transformation. Therefore Qi and Blood will move freely. Once again, Old Ten Needles formula emphasizes ZHONG WAN and ZU SAN LI. ZHONG WAN Adjusts the Middle and ZU SAN LI treats all the one hundred diseases. Therefore this formula can be used to treat other diseases (besides digestive disorders). For example, in post apoplectic hemiplegia, Old Ten Needles can commonly be added to shore up a course of treatment. It is especially indicated in hemiplegia with "dulled" Spleen and Stomach with irregular bowel or Bladder symptoms. In most cases, after one course (twelve treatments) with the original prescription (i.e. the specific needle prescription for the presenting symptoms), Old Ten Needles can be used for an additional six treatments. In normal situations where recovery is satisfactory, Old Ten Needles can be used until complete health is restored. For patients with hemiplegia, emaciated limbs and torso, and flaccid paralysis, based on the saying, "For flaccidity solely treat the Yang Ming", one can employ the Old Ten Needles to improve treatment efficacy.

For systemic Qi and Blood Deficiency with inability to grasp food, lack of harmony between Spleen and Stomach, fitful and easily disturbed sleep, and Heart palpitations, which includes the western diagnosis of neurasthenia, and the recurrence of chronic illness, employment of the Old Ten Needles in the treatment plan can help restore vigor and Calm the Mind. For paralysis due to external injury, the treatment is basically the same as for hemiplegia.

Menstual irregularities are usually disorders of the Qi and Blood. Among the Old Ten Needles SHANG WAN, ZHONG WAN, XIA WAN, and QI HAI are Ren Mai points. Moreover, ZHONG WAN is the Front MU point of the Stomach. There is the saying, "The Ren Mai is subdued under the Yang Ming." Thus, for patients with scanty menstrual flow due to Insufficient Qi and Blood, Blood Deficiency amenorrhea, or what could be summarized from experience as Deficient and Weak YUN HUA[3] of the Spleen and Stomach, the initial choice of treatment might very well be Old Ten Needles. Adjusting the Chong and Ren Mai through the Yang Ming is an ingenious treatment plan.

Old Ten Needles can also be used as an initial treatment for epilepsy by using ZHONG WAN and NEI GUAN as the primary points. This is especially effective in patients subject to epileptic seizures after eating or who have severe vomiting during a seizure. As for insertion depth for NEI GUAN, Dr. Wang counsels a relatively shallow insertion of approximately five FEN. Deep insertion should be avoided because this will exceed the meridian's depth and incur the effects of WAI GUAN. This point should be strictly noted.

OLD TEN NEEDLES MODIFICATIONS

When Dr. Wang Le-ting uses Old Ten Needles, he often makes alterations according to the patient's circumstances.

1) Delete SHANG WAN and XIA WAN and add ZHANG MEN (Liv 13)

This variation is called Old Excess Needles. The Chinese words for ten and Excess (SHI) are homonyms but obviously have different meanings. Old Excess Needles refers to Spleen Excess. ZHANG MEN is a point on the Foot Jue Yin Liver channel. It is the MU point of the Spleen and the meeting point of the ZANG. It is where Spleen Yin is stored. It is also where the Foot Jue Yin Liver channel meets the Foot Shao Yang Gallbladder channel. It Dredges the Liver and Promotes the Qi. When the Liver Qi is properly channelled, the Spleen and Stomach can find harmony. When the Liver and Spleen (Stomach) work together, the occurence of Qi's creation and transformation is just like a spring continuously gushing forth.

Usually it is thought that getting Qi to "Communicate" is a species of tonification, as is Activating the Blood. Dr. Wang adds ZHANG MEN to Adjust Liver and Spleen, Dredge the Qi and Blood, Tonify the Spleen, and Benefit the Qi. Since Old Ten Needles evolved from PI WEI LUN'S BU ZHONG YI QI formula it is not only indicated for symptoms due to Disharmony between the Liver and Stomach but also for Stuck Liver and Stagnant Qi, Liver Qi Crossing Over and Invading the Stomach, abdominal distention, intercostal neuralgia, nausea and vomiting, stomachaches with a sour taste, and other such symptoms. The prescription's principal points are ZHONG WAN, ZHANG MEN, and ZU SAN LI which all combine to Dredge the Liver and Promote the Qi, Ascend the Pure and Descend the Turbid, and Tonify the Middle and Benefit the Qi. Its most important indications are for treating constitutional weakness, Insufficient Middle Yang, exhaustion from over exertion, excess resting but failure to recuperate, and other signs of weakness and Deficiency. Using ZHONG WAN, ZHANG MEN, and ZU SAN LI as primary points, moxabustion on ZHONG WAN will Warm the Middle and disperse Cold, while ZHANG MEN Relaxes the Liver and Benefits the Spleen. Thus these points combine to Tonify the Middle and Benefit the Qi and Warm the Middle and Disperse Cold. Over time it will Correct and Solidify the Root.

2) Old Ten Needles with GUAN YUAN (CV 4) and SAN YIN JIAO (Sp 6)

Tonifying the Middle and Benefitting the Qi, Warming the Middle and Dispersing

Cold, and Adjusting and Promoting the Stomach and Intestines are all (principles) indicated for treating Deficiency Cold of the Spleen and Stomach, Cold Pathogen Attacking the Middle, or excessive eating which leads to Coldness and Cold abdominal pain. ZHONG WAN and ZU SAN LI are again the primary points. Tonifying ZHONG WAN strengthens the Stomach Qi and Disperses the Cold Pathogen. Dispersal of ZU SAN LI makes the Stomach Qi move downward, Descends the Turbid, and Drains Stagnation. When assisted by SHANG WAN and XIA WAN, it Settles the Stomach and Strengthens the Spleen. In combination with TIAN SHU, Turbid Qi of the abdomen is eliminated. Tonifying QI HAI Stabilizes the Yang Qi of the Lower Burner. Moxabustion on GUAN YUAN Warms and Disperses Cold Pathogen. Tonifying SAN YIN JIAO Tonifies the Liver, Spleen, and Kidney channels and these three in turn circulate the (lower) abdomen. By dredging these three channels they are open and pain-free.

3) Old Ten Needles with NEI TING (St 44)

Tonification of the Middle and Benefitting Qi while simultaneously Eliminating Food and Draining Stagnation are the requisite principles for treating Stagnant Food and Water, Stomach and Intestines Losing Control of Transportation, Non-separation of Clear and Turbid, and Obstructed Qi mechanism with symptoms such as stomachache, abdominal pain, nausea, halitosis, diarrhea with tenesmus, and pain that decreases after defecation. NEI TING is the YING Spring point of the Foot Yang Ming Stomach channel. Its functions are to Open and Descend the Stomach Qi, Harmonize the Intestines, and Transform Stagnation. Combined with Old Ten Needles, it strengthens the functions of Eliminating Food and Draining Stagnation.

4) Delete SHANG WAN, XIA WAN,and NEI GUAN; add GUAN YUAN, QU GU (CV 2), and SAN YIN JIAO

This formula is recommended for Blood Stagnation amenorrhea or for dysmenorrhea with Excess symptoms. Among the points, QU GU is a Ren Mai point that Tonifies the Kidneys and Strengthens the Yang, stops leukorrhea, and treats urination. SAN YIN JIAO Adjusts and Promotes the Spleen and Stomach and Separates and treats Damp Heat. When combined with GUAN YUAN and QI HAI, it Adjusts and Promotes the Ren Mai, Promotes the Qi, and Harmonizes the Blood. The complete prescription combines to Strengthen the Spleen, Tonify the Kidneys, Activate the Blood, Move the Qi, and stop pain.

SHI QUAN DA BU TANG & ACUPUNCTURE

SHI QUAN DA BU TANG (Ten Ingredients Major Tonification Decoction) is a Chinese medical prescription from the YI XUE FA MING. It consists of BA ZHEN TANG (Eight Pearls Decoction)[4] plus Astragalus and Cinnamon. Its purpose is to Tonify and Benefit both the Qi and the Blood. It is also indicated for Deficiency exhaustion with wheezing and coughing, spermatorrhea, hemorrhage, menorrhagia, and other menstrual irregularities. Dr. Wang believes that Traditional Chinese Medical theory is very important in the clinical application of acupuncture. To duplicate this famous classical prescription (with acupuncture), he selected several points which give in combination the same effect. SHI QUAN DA BU TANG is only one of the herbal formulae he has done this with.

SHI QUAN DA BU TANG includes the Qi-tonifying herbs Codonopsis, Poria,

Atractylodes, and Licorice and the Blood-tonifying herbs Cnidium, Tang Kuei, Cooked Rehmannia, and Peony. In addition, Sweet and Warming Raw Astragalus as well as Cinnamon for Warming the Kidneys and Assisting the Yang are included. This Tonifies both the Kidneys and the Spleen and aids both Yin and Yang. Therefore its tonifying effect is fairly strong.

Dr. Wang's needle prescription consists of the following points: HE GU (LI 4), QU CHI (LI 11), NEI GUAN, ZU SAN LI, YANG LING QUAN (GB 34), ZHONG WAN, TAI CHONG (Liv 3), SAN YIN JIAO, ZHANG MEN, and GUAN YUAN.

It is easily seen that this is a modification of (Dr. Wang's) Hand-Foot Twelve Needles formula[5]. In fact, it takes the original twelve needles and adds the MU point of the Spleen (ZHANG MEN), the MU point of the Stomach (ZHONG WAN), the MU point of the Small Intestine (GUAN YUAN), and the YUAN Source point of the Liver (TAI CHONG). Its functions are to Tonify the Qi and Blood, Strengthen the Spleen and Stomach, Nourish the Heart Qi, and Moisten the Liver and Kidneys while at the same time Openning the the JING (channels) and Activating the LUO (collaterals). Hand-Foot Twelve Needle formula tends to Dredge and Regulate, while SHI QUAN DA BU TANG (needle formula) tends to Regulate and Tonify.

ZHANG MEN is added to Tonify the Five ZANG[6], Settle the JING SHEN[7], Open the Heart and Benefit Wisdom, eliminate distention, and Transform Stagnant Food. In short, it has the same effects as Ginseng.[8] ZU SAN LI Rids Wind, Cold, and Damp BI[9], can Ascend or Descend, stops sweating and eliminates fever, Strengthens the Spleen, and Eliminates Stagnant Food. It has the same effects as Atractylodes. NEI GUAN Lowers Rebellious Qi from the thorax, Moves Qi and Blood, stops pain and congestion below the Heart, rids irritation and fullness, Strengthens the Spleen, and treats Dampness. It has the same effects as Poria. ZHONG WAN governs the Five ZANG and the Six FU, Solidifies the tendons and bones, helps muscle development, increases the Qi and Blood, and Adjusts Yin and Yang. It has the same effects as Licorice. SAN YIN JIAO governs irregular menstruation, Creates and Nourishes the Blood, stops Rebellious Qi of coughing, and governs the three Foot Yin meridians. Its effects are the same as Tang Kuei. QU CHI is indicated for ZHONG FENG[10], Cold BI, spasms, and amenorrhea. It especially Rids Wind from the Blood. Its effects are the same as Cnidium's. TAI CHONG governs Pathogenic Qi Damaging Yin, stops abdominal pain, Moves Blood and BI, Eliminates Stagnations, Enters the Jue Yin and Shao Yin, and treats Yin Deficiency dysuria. Its effects are the same as Peony's. GUAN YUAN treats Damaged Uterus due to Stagnant Blood, creates new Blood, builds bone and Marrow, and helps muscle development. It has the same effects as Rehmannia. HE GU treats Deficient WEI QI, Dredges and Opens the channels and collaterals, and enters the Tai Yin to either stop or induce sweating. It achieves similar effects as Astragalus. YANG LING QUAN governs cough from Rebellious Qi, Tonifies the Middle and Benefits Qi, Rids Wind, Cold, and Damp BI, and Relaxes tendons and treats the joints. It achieves similar effects as Cinnamon.

Using needles to stimulate acupuncture points based on their Chinese herbal characteristics and thereby creating a formula in this way is certainly a wondrous achievement.[11] Therefore, creating the SHI QUAN DA BU needle prescription from the original herbal formula fully and clearly shows Dr. Wang Le-ting's use and emphasis of basic TCM theory. This is the hallmark of his unique creation of acupuncture treatments.

In clinical use, SHI QUAN DA BU TANG is indicated in the treatment of Deficiency Damage symptoms. These can be summarized in the following few types:

1) Insufficient Qi and Blood with concomitant Heart and Spleen Deficiency

Usually such damage is due to extreme exhaustion or to too much thinking damaging the Spleen. It can also be caused by a chronic illness eliminating nourishment and damaging YUAN QI with injury reaching to the Heart and Spleen. And it can also be caused by excessive Blood loss in cases where it is difficult to create sufficient Qi and Blood. The most important manifestations (of this pattern) are shortness of breath, disinclination to speak, feeble voice, loss of appetite, diarrhea, dizziness, spontaneous sweating, palpitations, and numbness in the hands and feet. The tongue is pale and the pulse is deep, fine, and weak.

2) Spleen and Kidney Damaged; Pre and Postnatal lack of sustenance

Usually this is due to Congenital Deficiency, Postnatal lack of nurturing and wasting due to chronic illness, sexual excess, Prolapse of Middle Qi, or Unstable Kidney. The most important manifestations (of this pattern) are eating sparsely and Grasping inefficiently, emaciation and weakness, Exhausted Spirits, low back pain, dizziness, tinnitus, diarrhea, and polyuria. The tongue is pale and the pulse is deficient and weak.

3) Kidney Liver (Yin) Deficiency

This is usally due to the frailty of old age, Kidney Jing Damaged or Exhausted, wasting due to chronic illness, or after a high fever that results in damaged Liver and Kidney Yin. The most important manifestations are dizziness and vertigo, slight fever of the Five Hearts[12], a troubled Heart which is easily agitated, sore lower back, "jumping" legs[13], and polyuria. The pulse is fine and fast. The tongue is red with scant coating.

From the above explanations we can easily see that clinical use (of this formula) includes the treatment of neurasthenia, chronic, debilitating diseases, chronic illness in patients of weak constitution, and various geriatric diseases. Therefore, in the treatment of symptoms due to Deficiency and Damage or as a preventive treatment for older patients this formula has definite value.

THE SPECIAL CHARACTERISTICS OF GOLDEN NEEDLES

Wang Le-ting's gold needles and the gold needles mentioned in ancient sources have their differences. Ancient books refer to all needles made out of metal as "gold" needles. ZHEN JIU DA CHENG, for example, says, "Of old, gold needles are said to be valuable, but gold is just the common name. Copper, iron, gold, and silver are used as well." ZHEN JIU JING CUI says, "What the ancients called gold needles were not made of gold. This was a term of respect." The needles used by Wang Le-ting are an alloy of nine parts yellow gold and one part brass. This produces a needle different from silver, steel, or other metals. According to Wang Le-ting's experience, gold, silver, copper, and iron are all usable for making needles, but in the literature, needles made from gold are the most magnificent. When treating with gold needles the patients' spirits get a boost. Moreover, gold needles do not run hot and cold with seasonal changes. They match the (patient's) body temperature. They cause less pain on insertion. Once inserted they do not change; so there are no side effects and no trouble withdrawing them. The sites of insertion do not get infected and the curative response to them is quicker. They get high results, and because gold is soft they do not break easily. These characteristics (of true golden needles) have been summarized from (Wang Le-ting's) years of clinical experience.

WANG LE-TING'S STEP BY STEP PROTOCOL FOR LOCATING POINTS

Rubbing is the first step in locating a point. According to the position of the point, one should press and rub in the direction of the meridian flow. Especially in points on the four limbs, one should be sure to palpate all the muscles and joints in the area. This relaxes and opens the channels while simultaneously allowing the patient to prepare mentally. At the same time it allows the doctor to make a close inspection of the local area and the patient's body in general.

"Fingering" the point itself is commonly called "pinching the point". (This is the second step in Wang Le-ting's protocol.) After rubbing the general area, the next step is to locate the specific point on the meridian. Dr. Wang's method of point location is according to the traditional relationships of the bones and surface anatomy landmarks in particular area of the body. This is the way most texts commonly describe point locations. However, in a few cases, he has his own location method, such as for HUAN TIAO (GB 30), SAN JIAN (Three Shoulder points, i.e. JIAN YU (LI 15), JIAN LIAO (TH 14), and JIAN NEI LING), DU BI (St 35), etc. After finding the point, he uses the thumbnail of the left hand to draw a cross on the point such that the point of intersection of the two lines lies directly over the heart of the point. Finally he presses with his finger. Usually the patient will confirm that it is sore or distended.

On the one hand, this fingering method marks the site of insertion. On the other, palpation of the skin and muscle in the area numbs the site a bit and reduces pain on insertion. It also scatters the local Qi and Blood thus avoiding damage to the YING and WEI. After locating the point thus, one should next carry out standard antiseptic procedures.

Inserting the needle is the third step. After decades of clinical experience in inserting needles, Dr. Wang consistently uses both hands and is opposed to one-handed insertion. He emphasizes the importance of guiding with the left hand. He feels that with two-handed insertion the strength is appropriate, the needle is steady, the point is needled precisely, and there is no way to swing to the right or left nor movement up or down to cause the needle to miss its mark. Usually the patient feels no pain this way. As it says in the BIAO YOU FU, "The left hand is heavy and pressing down. This tends to lead the Qi towards dispersing. The right hand is light and moves quickly. This is the reason for no pain." All the time, while inserting, applying hand technique[14], and moving the needle, (Dr. Wang) always strictly follows the rules of protocol according to SU WEN, "ZHEN JIE PIAN": "The hand is as if grasping a tiger and admiring its strength. The Mind cares not for who or what is around. With a settled Will observing the patient, one looks neither to the right nor left."

THE NECESSITY OF USING TONIFICATION & DISPERSAL HAND TECHNIQUES

After the needle has been inserted and achieved DE QI[15], a hand technique should be immediately employed, but also not over-employed. According to SU WEN, "ZHEN JIE PIAN", "When the meridian Qi has arrived, the good doctor holds it without losing it and avoids surprising changes." Dr. Wang strongly emphasizes using hand technique on every single insertion. Though there are many hand techniques in acupuncture and they all have their good points, Dr. Wang uses only dispersion of Excess and tonification of Deficiency techniques. He leaves all the rest alone. He feels that man is a unified, complete system and that one should maintain balance in the opposites of Yin and Yang.

If a pathogen invades or if any of the Six Qi[16] becomes established internally, Yin and Yang lose their balance and disease occurs. As for Excess and Deficiency, the SU WEN, "TONG PING XU SHI LUN" records, "A flourishing Pathogenic Qi is Excess and Jing or Qi released is Deficiency." Once a disease has set in, it can be none other than Excess, Deficiency, or a combination of the two. According to the principle, "If Deficient, tonify. If Excess, disperse", for Deficiency symptoms one should tonify and for Excess, disperse. For combinations of the two, the Deficiencies should be given tonification, while the Excesses should be dispersed. Logically there is no such thing as neither Excess nor Deficient, for in that case Yin and Yang would be balanced, the patient would be normal, and there would be no need for acupuncture. Therefore, in hand technique there should never be a situation requiring "even technique"[17]. To tonify is to tonify. To dipserse is to disperse. The use of tonification and dispersal should be strictly divided. Of course, in tonification and dispersion the patient's individual situation should be taken into account regarding the strength of stimulation. (Rejecting) the so-called "neither Deficient nor Excess, just let the meridian take care of it" (i.e. Even method), Dr. Wang Le-ting thinks that (through the proper hand technique) DE QI can be improved and that this difference allows one to accomplish their aim.

Because the direction of flow is different on the left and right sides, tonification and dispersal techniques are different as well. For example, in tonifying the Hand Yang Ming point HE GU, when needling the left side one should move the thumb backwards and the index finger forwards so that the needle twirls to the left (Counterclockwise). Needling HE GU on the right side, one's thumb should move forward and index finger backwards so that the needle twirls to the right (clockwise). In order to disperse, the opposite should be done. For arms and legs, right and left, tonification and dispersion, the following chart is offered to simplify and explain.

MERIDIANS:		HAND YANG	FOOT YIN	HAND YIN	FOOT YIN	REN & DU
Direction of Flow		Hand to Head	Foot to Abdomen	Chest to Hand	Head to Foot	Circling
Tonification	L	Counterclockwise		Clockwise		Clockwise
	R	Clockwise		Counterclockwise		
Dispersal	L	Clockwise		Counterclockwise		Counter-clockwise
	R	Counterclockwise		Clockwise		

In summary, amongst the twelve meridians, the three Hand Yang and the three Foot Yin use the same hand techniques as do the three Hand Yin and three Foot Yang. The Conception Vessel and Governing Vessel also share the same techniques. Man responds to the interplay of Heaven and Earth. "Earth Qi rises to form the clouds. Heaven Qi descends as rain." Heaven is Yang and Earth is Yin. Yin Qi ascends and Yang Qi descends. From the workings of man's Qi mechanism we can say that the left ascends and the right descends. Therefore, Yin meridians should be raised to tonify and descended to disperse. Yang meridians should be descended to tonify and raised to disperse. In short, going in the direction of the meridian and stimulating the needle is tonifying, while going against the meridian is dispersing.

Dr. Wang works strictly according to where the fourteen meridians arise and their direction of flow as well as the (above-mentioned) Ascending the Yin/Descending the Yang rationale to carry out tonification and dispersion. When the selection of light, medium, or heavy manipulation is added, it completes an easy to perform method that achieves good results in tonifying Deficiency and dispersing Excess. He rarely uses or supports other fancy hand techniques or tries to explore other systems. Rather, he consistently diagnoses according to Deficiency and Excess and clearly separates whether to tonify or disperse as well as how much stimulation to use.

As for removing the needle, (Dr. Wang) also does not let this go unnoticed. As it is said in SU WEN, "ZHEN JIE PIAN", "When Evil Qi is victorious, then empty it. Remove the needle and do not cover it." When the pathogen is flourishing and the patient is exhibiting Excess symptoms, do not cover the hole. Rather, let the pathogen drain out. If the Righteous Qi is Deficient, then slowly remove the needle and quickly cover the hole thus allowing the Righteous Qi to fill in and avoiding any further damage from the outside. When removing the needle, first spin it a little in both directions to loosen the surrounding tissue. This avoids a stuck needle and prevents damage to the environ. Afterwards proceed according to the above instructions for either tonification or dispersion. One should try to start properly and finish properly making the treatment reach and maintain a plateau through a set period of time. To cultivate discipline, one should oppose the practice of withdrawing needles as if pulling onions.

HUN MEN (Bl 47) & PO HU (Bl 42)

HUN MEN and PO HU are both Foot Tai Yang Bladder meridian points that are adjacent to GAN SHU (Bl 18) and FEI SHU (Bl 13) (respectively). The Liver treasures HUN[18] and the Lungs treasure PO[19]. Moreover, the Liver treasures Blood and the Lungs govern Qi. If Qi and Blood are not regulated, then PO and HUN do not communicate. This develops into Heart agitation causing unpeaceful SHEN and Will, insomnia, and disturbing dreams. Foot Tai Yang Bladder meridian rules the Exterior and unites the entire body's Qi. Each of the ZANG-FU connect with Tai Yang and their SHU points are all located on the back. Because they all connect with the Tai Yang Bladder meridian, it acts like the sun's beams in warming and shining which thus adjusts the QI HUA function and makes the Qi and Blood settled and peaceful.

Thus combining PO HU and HUN MEN Adjusts the Qi and Blood while Settling the Heart and SHEN. It Rectifies the HUN and Settles the PO. Clinically it can be combined with SHEN MEN (Ht 7) with dispersion technique to clear the Heart and Settle the SHEN, or with SAN YIN JIAO with tonification technique to Nourish the Blood and Rectify the Liver. This brings good results.

FOR HIGH BLOOD PRESSURE

Based on the differentiation of Excess and Deficiency, use appropriate tonification and dispersion techniques. For Yin Deficient/Yang Rebelling hypertension, use tonification on the Yin JING Stream points and dispersion on the Yang JING Stream points. With time, their Yin and Yang will become harmonized. For dizziness, add BAI HUI (GV 20). For difficulty speaking, add LIAN QUAN (CV 23). For Phlegm with Fire or Liver Fire Rising, use dispersion technique with Hand-Foot Twelve Needle formula. For Phlegm, add TIAN TU (CV 22) and ZHONG WAN. For anger with headache, use TAI CHONG to disperse Liver-Gallbladder Fire.

ENDNOTES

1 Li Dong-Yuan was one of the Four Great Masters of Internal Medicine (i.e. herbalism) of the Jin-Yuan dynasties. The PI WEI LUN is his great masterpiece upon which the BU TU PAI (School of Tonifying Earth) is founded. This is primarily an herbal as opposed to an acupuncture text.

2 QI HUA: literally Energy Transformation. This refers to the Qi's function as the energy initiating and carrying out metabolic transformations. In a narrower sense it usually refers to the Qi's transforming or metabolizing liquids.

3 YUN HUA means Transportation and Transformation.

4 Ingredients of BA ZHEN TANG according to Yeung Him-che in Handbook of Chinese Herbs and Formulas, (LA 1983) Vol. 2, p.33

Cooked Rehmannia
Tang Kuei
Peony
Cnidium
Ginseng
Atractylodes
Poria
Zizyphus sattiva
Baked Licorice
Fresh Ginger

5 Dr. Wang Le-ting's Hand-Foot Twelve Needle formula: HE GU, NEI GUAN, QU CHI, SAN YIN JIAO, ZU SAN LI, YANG LING QUAN

6 Five ZANG: the five primary "organs" of Chinese medicine. These are the Heart, Liver, Spleen, Lungs, and Kidneys. However, as Manfred Porkert and Ted Kaptchuk point out, these are not identical with the western biological organs of the same name. They are physiological concepts which have no identical western counterparts.

7 JING SHEN: spirit or mood. It is the manifestation of the configurative force.

8 In daily practice, Codonopsis is usually substituted in formulae which call for Ginseng. It has most of the same properties without being so expensive.

9 BI: obstruction to the flow of Qi and Blood in one or more meridians.

10 ZHONG FENG: stroke or apoplexy due to Internal Wind

11 This is a controversial point. Does acupuncture indeed work in the same manner as herbal therapy? Should both modalities be based on a single theory or approach?

12 Five Hearts: the center of the chest, the palms of the hands, and the soles of the feet. A feverish sensation felt in all or some of these indicates Yin Deficiency.

13 Jumping legs: this refers either to muscle spasm, muscular twitching, or formication.

14 Hand technique: specific manipulations of the needle after insertion designed to achieve specific alterations in the energy. Classical hand techniques often have such fancy and allusive names as Green Dragon Wagging its Tail, etc.

15 DE QI: Arrival of the Qi. This is characterised by the patient's subjective sensations of soreness, distention, heaviness, or tingling at the point after insertion and objectively by the feel of resistance of the needle in the acupuncturist's fingers.

16 Six Qi: Wind, Hot, Cold, Damp, Dryness, and Summer Heat

17 Even technique: in contemporary Chinese acupuncture this refers to refraining from employing any particular tonification or dispersal hand techniques after DE QI has been achieved.

18 HUN: one of the psychophysical constituents of the bodymind. It is sometimes translated as soul. It is stored in the Liver and is associated with thinking.

19 PO: another of the psychophysical constituents of the bodymind. This is the animal or vegetative sould which returns to the Earth upon death. It is associated with the physique and with physical vigor.

OF BABIES & BATHWATER

A Critical Examination of Zhang Zi-he And the Implications of His Theories on Modern Healthcare

One of Chinese medicine's greatest assets is its unbroken clinical and literary history of no less than two thousand years. In each generation since the Han dynasty, eminent physicians have summed up their life's work and practical experience in written texts and oral instructions bequeathed to their students. Over the centuries many different medical theories and therapies were propounded. Some of these were verified in clinical practice by succeeding generations of doctors. These have come down to us today as the generally accepted guiding principles of Chinese medicine. Other theories and therapies were modified by succeeding generations in an effort to improve them in the light of their clinical experience. And yet others were found to be erroneous, ineffective, or even deleterious in the long run. The history of classical Chinese medicine is not the story of a single homogeneous theory or a single orthodox practice. Its theory and practice continue to develop today, contrary to some writers' opinions.[1]

As contemporary practitioners of classical Chinese medicine constantly trying to improve upon our abilities and techniques as healers, we can and should look back at what has been tried in the past and been found to be ineffective or detrimental and avoid such mistakes in our own practice. This is especially necessary today when a welter of "new" or "alternative" theories and therapies are being marketed to an increasingly health conscious public. From Chinese medicine's two thousand year perspective, most of these therapies are not, in fact, new and we can go back to the classics to see how these therapies fared over generations in the past. In this way we can learn from our medical forebears' mistakes and save ourselves and our patients time, energy, money, and the precious treasure of health.

As mentioned in a previous essay, there were four great schools of Internal medicine of the Jin-Yuan dynasties. Each of these schools is associated with the name of a preeminent doctor. Liu Wan-su was the founder of the School of Cool and Cold (Medicine). Li Dong-yuan was the founder of the School of Stomach/Spleen. And Zhu Dan-xi was the founder of the School of Watering

Yin. But the name of the founder of the fourth school is hardly remembered by anyone. In fact, this fourth physician's theory and practice turned out to be so weak in comparison to those of the three above-named doctors that in the Ming dynasty Zhang Zhung-jing's name was substituted instead.[2] It was not until the Qing dynasty that the name Zhang Zi-he was restored to its proper historical place.[3]

During Zhang Zi-he's lifetime he and his students believed that his theory of medicine was adequate to describe and treat all pathologies. Zhang Zi-he's method is known as the School of Attacking and Purging. Zhang believed "that all diseases, whether from internal or external causes, are manifestations of evil ch'i. To effect a cure, the physician must purge the evil ch'i. In his therapeutic treatise he describes three methods of attacking and purging: sweating, vomiting, and purging. Although these three methods originated in the SHAN HAN LUN, (Zhang) revised the theories to make the therapy more widely applicable. He claimed that these three methods included all therapeutic techniques."[4]

In classical Chinese medicine Evil Qi (XIE QI) is defined in juxtaposition to Righteous Qi. Righteous Qi are all the energies and pure substances which are appropriate to the body and its functions. These include WEI QI, YING QI, XUE, YUAN QI, JIN-YE, ZONG QI, etc. Evil Qi are all energies and substances in the body which are pathologic or pathogenic. These include the invasion of the Six Cosmopathogenic energies, internally produced Stagnant Qi, Stagnant Blood, Stagnant Fluid, Stagnant Food, Phlegm, Toxins (DU), and transformative pathologic Heat.

Over the centuries, Chinese medicine has developed two broad categories of therapy. One is tonification or support of the Righteous Qi. The other is the dispersal of Evil Qi. Emesis, diaphoresis, and purgation are the three basic methods (SAN FA) of dispersal according to Zhang Zi-he. All three of these methods, however, result not only in the dispersal of the Evil Qi but also in the inevitable loss of some of the patient's Righteous Qi in the process. For instance, sweating disperses the WEI QI and Fluid thus weakening the Yin and YING as well as expelling any pernicious invading energies lodged in the WEI or superficial layer. Likewise, vomiting and purgation disperse the Middle Qi and Fluid thus weakening all the Post Natal Qi.

In patients whose pathology is described in Chinese medicine as a simple Excess imposed upon a strong constitution, the employment of one of these three methods may be an appropriate therapy. However, in patients whose pathology is an Excess superimposed upon a Deficient constitution, employment of these three methods may lead to iatrogenic complications. In such cases which are a mixed type of simultaneous Excess and Deficiency, one must assess the relative strength and weakness of the Evil and Righteous Qi and decide whether to 1) attack the Evil first and then later tonify the Righteous, 2) tonify the Righteous first and later attack the Evil, or 3) to tonify and attack simultaneously. In cases of simple Deficiency, dispersal is contraindicated categorically. In such cases the symptoms of disease are due to a decline in vital function and exhausted substance and are not due to the presence of an Evil Qi.

This descrimination of the relative importance of attacking the Evil and supporting the Righteous is one of the great treasures of Chinese medicine. By and large, western allopathic medicine pays scant attention to the support of the patient's Righteous Qi. It is focused almost entirely on and excels at attacking the Evil in the form of bacteria, viruses, neoplasms, etc. Just as many Americans are turning from western allopathic care because of its iatrogenic complications due to its overemphasis on heroic attack, so the generations of Chinese doctors and patients following Zhang Zi-he quickly saw that his emphasis on attacking the Evil was not adequate to treat the complexity of most disease, especially chronic disease.[4] Subsequent generations have established that Zhang's three methods, although necessary and useful in some cases, need to be seen as only a part of the classical Eight Methods (PA FA). These include calorification, refrigeration, tonification, harmonizing, and dispersion in addition to emesis, diaphoresis, and purgation. The importance of assessing the relative proportions of attacking and supporting in erecting a treatment plan is clearly exemplified by the following case history.

A thirty-five year old man had had chronic diarrhea for one year. He was fatigued, emaciated, listless, and chilled. He also had thrush in his mouth and herpes zoster on his chest. He had recently recieved a western diagnosis of Autoimmune Deficiency Syndrome (AIDS). When he was brought to me he could not walk, looked grey and cadaverous, and was also vomiting and hiccoughing. His pulse was slow, sunken, and minute. He had been hospitalized for some time and had been given large doses of antibiotics for the diarrhea and the thrush but to no avail. It was immediately apparent to me that support of the Righteous was more important than attacking the Evil as the western allopaths were doing with their antibiotics. I made regulation of the digestion with cessation of vomiting and diarrhea and restoration of the body warmth my first priorities. My prescription for this patient was ZHEN WU TANG.[5] I also taught the patient's sister how to administer indirect moxabustion at ZU SAN LI (St 36), ZHONG WAN (CV 12), GUAN YUAN (CV 4), and PI SHU (Bl 20) and explained the principles of a warming, tonifying diet according to the theory of Li Dong-yuan. My treatment plan was to first tonify the Righteous Qi and then to eventually simultaneously attack the Evil Toxins with LIU SHEN WAN or some other such medicine.

After approximately one week the patient reported a cessation of vomiting and hiccoughs. His diarrhea was also markedly diminished as were his chills. He also reported a slight return of energy. Unfortunately those around him had difficulties understanding and carrying out the administration of his herbs, moxabustion, and diet. A "friend" brought the patient some marijuana brownies which he ate and immediately thereafter began vomiting and having diarrhea again. Cannabis seeds are considered a purgative and cannabis leaves exhaust the MING MEN HUO. Scared, the patient readmitted himself to the hospital. There the doctors would not allow him to continue receiving Chinese herbal medicine nor would they allow moxabustion due to its smell and the hospital smoke alarms. The patient was put back on antibiotics and died several months later without ever leaving the hospital. Although AIDS is considered currently incurable by western clinicians, it can be clearly described in Chinese medicine as a mixed Deficiency/Toxic pattern of disharmony and theoretically should be treatable by Chinese medicne.[6] In my opinion, this patient's death is to some extent attributable to a lack of understanding of the importance of supporting the Righteous and effective methods to accomplish that on the part of his doctors.

However, on the contemporary scene it is not only the allopaths who are guilty of committing Zhang Zi-he's mistake of overemphasizing the attack of the Evil. A large proportion of so-called alternative healthcare practitioners also operate either consciously or unconsciously on the assumption that all disease is due to Evil Qi. The common term is "toxins", a concept which is not the same as that of Toxins in classical Chinese medicine and which, in general, is only loosely defined by most western practitioners. This particular concept of toxicity originates in the late nineteenth century. The great Nobel Prize-winning biologist, Elie Metchnikoff, questioning why humans rarely live to one hundred years of age, introduced the notion that degenerative disease in general is due to intestinal putrefaction with attendant autotoxicity.[7] This idea seems to have found more favor with the naturopaths of his day than with the allopaths who were drunk on the idea that there was a specific germ as the cause of each and every disease. According to modern usage, toxins may be metabolic by-products retained within the body rather than being eliminated through normal channels, i.e. the bowels, skin, breath, or urine, or may be external environmental pollutants which accumulate in the body. In either case, this accumulation leads to an impairment of the healthy functioning of the body and the production of disease. The symptoms of disease are seen from this point of view as an expression of the body's own attempts to discharge these toxins. The following quotes from a selection of different writers whose books are sold in American health food stores underscore the belief that all disease is due to toxicity, in Chinese terms Evil Qi, and that the best therapy for the restoration of health is the discharge or dispersal of these toxins.

Arnold Ehret, the father of the "mucousless" diet, states: "Every disease, no matter what name it is known by Medical Science, is Constipation, a clogging up of the entire pipe system of the body. Any special symptom is therefore merely an extraordinary local constipation by more accumulated mucous at this particular place."[8] Norman W. Walker states: "The fact of the matter is that constipation is the number one affliction underlying nearly every ailment; it can be imputed to be the initial, primary cause of nearly every disturbance of the human system."[9] Bernard Jensen writes: "In the 50 years I've spent helping people overcome illness, disability, and disease, it has become crystal clear that poor bowel management lies at the root of most people's health problems...I believe autointoxication is currently the number one source of the misery and decay we are witnessing in our society and culture today."[10] Dr. Jensen goes on to say, "Detoxification is often neglected, overlooked, or underestimated in the healing arts, despite the fact that all health professionals realize that a sick body is a toxic body...When these (toxins) can be eliminated from the body, there is no problem... I am convinced that toxic accumulations in the body create the necessary preconditions for disease to develop."[11] Stanley Burroughs makes the same statement even more boldly: "For the novice and the advanced student alike, cleansing is basic for the elimination of every kind of disease. The purpose of this book (THE MASTER CLEANSER) is to simplify the cause and the correction of all disorders, regardless of name or names. As we eliminate and correct one disease, we correct them all, for every disease is corrected by the same process of cleansing..."[12] And finally, J.H. Tilden writes: "In a few words: Without Toxemia there can be no disease. I knew that the waste-product of metabolism was toxic and that the only reason why we were not poisoned by it was because it was removed from the organism as fast as produced. Then I decided that the toxin was retained in the blood, when there was a checking of elimination. Eureka! the cause of all so-called disease is found. Ennervation checks the elimination of the waste-products of metabolism. Retention of metabolic toxin -- the first and only cause of disease!"[13] Tilden even elevates this theory to the status of philosophy. "According to Toxin Philosophy, every so-called disease is a crisis of Toxemia; which means that toxin has accumulated in the blood above the toleration point, and the crisis, the so-called disease -- call it cold, 'flu', pneumonia, headache, or typhoid fever -- is a vicarious elimination. Nature is endeavoring to rid the body of toxin. Any treatment that obstructs this effort at elimination baffles nature in her effort at self-curing."[14]

The major therapeutic modes logically derived from this theory as practised by western healers are fasting, purgation, and sweating. Fasting may be complete fasting supplemented only by water, the ingestion of a monofood diet such as certain types of juices, fruits, or brown rice, or a severely limited diet whose emphasis is on "cleansing" or "purification". According to this approach, if the therapy is successful it may provoke a "healing crisis". This is the temporary exacerbation of the symptoms followed by a rapid and complete recovery. If cleansing is continued, adherents believe that one can expel suppressed or latent toxins from old diseases. These latent toxins are often believed to be due to the iatrogenic complications of allopathic treatment. In such cases, the most recent diseases will be expelled first and the oldest last. This is according to Hering's Law of Cure, a statement of theory almost universally accepted by proponents of the toxin school of disease. Hering's Law states: "All cure starts from within out and from head down and in reverse order as the symptoms appeared."[15]

Although Metchnikoff is the probable theoretical founder of this theory of disease, Arnold Ehret, quoted above, is popularly regarded as the father of this school of thought. His book, THE MUCUSLESS DIET HEALING SYSTEM, first appeared in 1922. According to Ehret's particular perspective on toxemia, all disease is due to an accumulation of mucous. This mucous is produced in the digestive tract. Unlike Chinese medicine which emphasizes that mucous is primarily due to weak digestion and overeating in general and only secondarily to the inherent Dampness of certain foods, Ehret emphasized that certain foods intrinsically produce mucous. His list of mucous producing foods is a long one. Basically Ehret advocated a raw fruit and vegetable diet. He believed that if one eliminated all mucous-producing food from the diet the body would eventually cleanse itself of any old accumulations of mucous wherever these were lodged. In this process all symptoms due to an accumulation of mucous, whether local or systemic, would disappear. Even though Ehret wrote in an archaic Victorian style, his books are still reprinted and sell well in American healthfood stores.

Although there are numerous schools and therapies each with their own name which ascribe to this idea that all disease is due to toxemia, for simplicity's sake I refer to this general school of thought as naturopathy in contradistinction to allopathy. This term, I believe, includes not only Naturopathy as founded by Benjamin Lust but also the majority of contemporary alternative therapies. Even the quasi-Oriental theory of Macrobiotics seems to me to have more in common with naturopathy than with classical Chinese medicine. It is interesting to note that naturopathy developed in a milieu dominated by three intellectual trends. The first and most important was the zeitgeist of the Industrial Revolution. This was the belief in the independence of man from nature and, as a corollary, a belief in the technological imperative by which man can and should dominate nature. So-called scientific solutions were sought for all the problems of life including disease. This was called Progress and this concept fostered the notion that everything is fixable and subject to human manipulation. Such a notion is inherently aggressive and led to violence on every level as evidenced for instance by the rape of the environment and colonialism. This aggressiveness also fostered the notion that the treatment of disease is a battle or war.

The second trend was the Victorian Protestant revival with its emphasis on sin and purification. Mankind was seen as inherently sinful and a person had to be cleansed by the Holy Spirit in order to be saved from damnation. Since the wages of sin are death and concomitantly disease, illness was often accepted as a sign of pollution. This was also the era that espoused that cleanliness is next to Godliness. It was an age of starched white collars, white linen suits, virginity, and the purgation from "polite" conversation of all references to "unclean" bodily functions. It was a time when even underwear were unmentionable and it is not difficult to understand how such people might subconsciously crave a sqeaky-clean colon devoid of feces.

The third trend was the recent development of the germ theory of disease. Germs were touted as the ultimate cause of disease by the emerging allopaths who saw the job of healing as a battle against evil invaders. Once again the emphasis was on achieving antiseptic purity and the conquering and killing of pathogens. While the naturopaths rejected the idea that germs were the ultimate cause of disease, still they accepted an only slightly different version of this medical model in which illness is based on the presence of some Evil Qi. Whether the therapist believes that he must purify his patient from germs or from toxins is conceptually only a small difference.

In America these beliefs and trends met with the rigors of frontier life. Outside of the cities people were forced to depend on locally gathered herbs and self-administered therapies. Often these were borrowed from the indigenous Indian population, but, I suspect, without also adopting the conceptual framework used by the Indians. Rather these pioneers fit the symptomatic actions of these herbs into their own notions of health and disease based on such nineteenth century preoccupations as Original Sin, fighting Evil, purifications, etc. From this perspective, naturopathy is not different fundamentally from allopathy. Both are based on a similar medical model and theory of disease, i.e. that there is something bad inside which must be either killed or gotten out. The difference between naturopathy and allopathy is simply a difference in therapeutic methodology. Indeed, both systems adopt a physiology based on nineteenth and twentieth century western biology. If one talks with a naturopath or the majority of alternative healthcare practitioners, they all describe the structure and function of the human organism in terms of western anatomy and physiology. This definition of disease as being caused by toxins, or in Chinese terms Evil Qi, is essentially the same theory of disease as Zhang Zi-he's.

As a practitioner of Chinese medicine in America, I often see patients who, based on this pervasive notion of toxicity and discharge common to contemporary alternative healthcare, have made their situation worse instead of better. In PRINCE WEN HUI'S COOK I have written at length about the deleterious effects of excessive fasting, fruitarianism, and a raw food diet on many young Americans who have practiced these over a long period of time. Such therapies may have been appropriate for our more constitutionally robust and less stressed grandparents, but, by and large, they are not, in my opinion, healthy for long-term adherence by contemporary young adults. In "The Tale of the Red-tipped Tongue", I have discussed the stresses of our society and environment and the endemic Deficiency Heat these have produced. Since the majority of younger Americans suffer from mixed Excess/Deficiency patterns of disharmony as described by Chinese medicine, fasting, cleansing, and purgation are not the panaceas they are commonly touted to be. Although these methods are attractive because of their conceptual simplicity, our health problems today are a reflection of our increasingly complex world and demand more sophisticated conceptual remedies. The following case histories exemplify how the employment of an erroneous treatment principle based on a simplistic notion of discharge can cause ill health and complicate the treatment of an existing pattern of disharmony.

A woman 45 years old complained of continual constipation. She was considerably overweight and lacked muscle tone. Her face was slightly yellowish. She slept ten to twelve hours per night and woke up exhausted. Her blood pressure was low normal and she had had hemorrhoids for years. In the past these had sometimes bled but now they were not particularly painful. Her hands and feet were habitually cold. Her tongue was slightly pale with a white, slightly thick but not greasy coat. Her pulse was thready, sunken, and slightly wirey.

My Chinese diagnosis for this patient was Spleen Deficiency causing a breakdown in the YUN HUA function of the Middle and Lower Burners and the Stagnation of Liver Qi. A number of acupuncture treatments at ZHI GOU (TH 6), YANG LING QUAN (GB 34), TIAN SHU (St 25), and DA CHANG SHU (Bl 25) in combination with the Decoction for Warming the Spleen[16] produced absolutely no result. This woman had been involved with various types of healing over a period of ten years. She had tried many different types of diet, most of which were based on the concept of discharge and purification. She had also undergone a series of colonic irrigations to "cleanse her bowels". After <u>sixty</u> such treatments she could no longer have a bowel movement without recourse to various "natural" laxatives such as Cascara sagrada.

I switched the patient to a modified version of Tonifying the Center and Supporting the Qi Decoction. Its ingredients included:

Astragalus	8 grams
Atractylodes alba	8
Cimicifuga	2
Zizyphus sattiva	4
Codonopsis	8
Orange Peel	4
Bupleurum	4
Treated Licorice	3
Tang Kuei	6
Aconite	6
Rhubarb	7
Fresh Ginger	4 slices

The amount of Rhubarb in this formula had to be adjusted over a period of a couple of weeks. If the amount fell below 6 grams per BAO, the patient would not have a bowel movement. If the amount reached 9 grams per BAO, the patient experienced loose stools. Since this patient had a complication of Liver Qi Congestion, this formula with its inclusion of Bupleurum, Tang Kuei, and Orange Peel succeeded in keeping the patient's elimination regular. Whereas the first formula without ingredients to move the Liver failed. This patient has had to remain on this formula for several months. If she stops taking it her constipation returns. Although Chinese herbal therapy is not a dietary supplement to be taken forever, in this case, because of the patient's unskillful reliance on detoxifying therapies, she had severely weakened her Middle Burner Fire and it will take some time to restore this lost Qi. It is also because of the degree of weakness that the Liver-moving acupuncture was not effective. There was not enough Qi to tap with the needles to catalyse an effect. This patient was Spleen Deficient long before she received the sixty colonics as evidenced by her chronic cold hands and feet, obesity, constipation, and bleeding hemorrhoids. However, the extreme purgation of the colonics exhausted the Middle Burner Fire even more.

A somewhat similar case involved a 46 year old man. When he first came to me he just wanted an overall examination. His only complaints were fatigue and extreme flatulence. On questioning it turned out that his stools were consistently loose. These symptoms had begun six months previous after having a series of colonics. His tongue was reddish and cracked. His pulse was a bit slippery and wirey on the right and finer, weaker, and not slippery on the left. My diagnosis was Deficient Yin and Damp Spleen. This patient responded well to the following formula:

Coptis	3 grams
Donkey skin gelatin	9
Scutellaria	9
Peony	12
Ophiopogon	9
Dendrobium	9
Atractylodes	9
Orange Peel	6
Siler	9
One egg yolk	

In cases of Yin Deficiency there is the tendency for Dampness to accumulate due to the Qi becoming weak. Because of the connection between the Large Intestine, the Internal Duct of the Triple Heater, and the Kidney Yin, the Root of Yin, the purgation of the colonics probably exhausted the Yin further, tipping the balance towards Dampness in the Middle JIAO. This patient, using an erroneous treatment principle of purgation, caused himself months of less than vibrant health.

The last case involved a 35 year old woman. She had been diagnosed by an MD as having bronchitis. She had been sick for one month. Her phlegm was a thick, deep yellow sometimes flecked with blood. She had three bowel movements per day which were a little loose due to her self-administering megadoses of Vitamin C.

Her tongue was slightly red and fluted with a scant coat. Her pulse was superficial, finish, and slippery. My diagnosis was Phlegm Heat in the Lungs with underlying Yin Deficiency. She received acupuncture for three days in a row with needles inserted at FEI SHU (Bl 13), HE GU (LI 4), FENG LONG (St 40), LIE JUE (Lu 7), and CHI ZE (Lu 5). I also advised her not to take the Vitamin C and to avoid dairy products. Because this patient was a nutritional counselor she was heavily influenced by the theory of toxicity and discharge. After each acupuncture treatment she felt better but, trying to speed up her cure, she took a lengthy steam bath which completely exhausted her. Because of her underlying Yin Deficiency, the loss of sweat, rather than purging toxicity, resulted in her severely depleting her Righteous Qi. When criticized for her uninformed intervention, the patient became defensive and discontinued treatment. Left to her own devices, the patient continued being sick for another six weeks.

Patients often ask if they should fast in order to treat their problems. The idea of burning off or discharging toxins is a simple one. It is straight forward, uncomplicated, and appeals to our desire to find a solution to our problems which is a one step affair. What most of us want is to purify ourselves once and then live happily ever after, at least most of us who have grown up in a Judeo-Christian culture. However this is not a realistic approach to either health or life in general. There are no quick fixes. Any theory of disease which relies on only one concept cannot possibly account for all the various factors which produce so many different diseases in so many different individuals. Chinese medicine over the past two thousand years has seen such theories come and go.

Zhang Zi-he's School of Attacking and Purging has been proven by history to be incomplete. It is not that sweating, vomiting, and purgation are never appropriate but only that they are not always appropriate. In order to treat disease effectively we must always balance the attacking of Evil with the support of the Righteous. Both contemporary allopathy and most alternative healthcare methods derived from naturopathy could learn some valuable lessons from the history of Chinese medicine on this point.

On the other hand, in my experience, American practitioners of Traditional Chinese Medicine are not usually adequately trained in the use of Zhang's three methods. Because we are not called on to treat acute, infectious diseases with regularity, many of us do not keep this area of our knowledge and technique well honed. This can cause some difficulty in treating certain Stagnations such as are often involved in cancer. All too often we tend to look for a single formula, be it acupuncture or herbal, which will neutralize the situation in one step. Such formulae tend to be based on attacking and supporting simultaneously. However, in complicated cases such as cancer where there is usually mixed Excess/Deficiency, a several step, prioritized treatment plan is often necessary. Treatments that try to do everything at once often do nothing well. In a step-by-step treatment, each step must be based on a clear assessment of whether to tonify first and then disperse or to disperse first and then tonify. Simultaneously doing both, while appearing safe on paper, often does not work. Sometimes it is necessary to simply disperse based on the calculated risk.

Most of this essay has been written from the perspective of a negative critique of Zhang Zi-he's work. However Zhang did make some observations which are germane to another facet of healthcare in America. Due to our cultural bias, many Americans operate on a "more is better" principle. Based on this principle many Americans self-medicate themselves with megadoses of vitamins and take various tonics without an accurate assessment of their need. It is ironic that many Americans have perverted the use of Chinese herbal tonics. Such tonics are what western allopathic medicine largely lacks to support the Righteous Qi. However their indescriminate use itself causes many problems and may eventually supply fuel to those allopaths who are threatened by Chinese medicine. Zhang felt that tonics should not be taken unless the patient was clinically Deficient. In such cases, the nature of the Deficiency should be well delineated and just the proper tonic used to redress that particular weakness. Just yesterday I saw a young American man who was taking several Chinese tonic formulae. Each day of the week he took a different tonic to "strenghten" a different organ or system. In actual fact, what this man needed was the dispersal of Internal Heat and cooling of the Blood. Zhang felt that the average person, like this patient, should not resort to tonics as a means of some sort of superhealth but that they should maintain good health primarily through a well-balanced and adjusted diet and lifestyle. If more energy is generated than can be circulated adequately, it will cause stagnation. Many tonic herbs also cause Dampness to accumulate internally, thus obstructing digestion. Stagnation of Qi or Blood or Dampness and Phlegm are complications which only make subsequent treatment more difficult. Phlegm and Dampness are especially recalcitrant to treatment since they impede the herbal ingredients from getting into the system. Zhang's criticism of the indescriminate use of tonics is worthy of popularization at this time when all sorts of tonics are being marketed in healthfood and drugstores capitalizing on peoples' insecurity and the mystique of the East.

Zhang Zi-he, in his major work, HOW TO ATTEND THE FAMILY (JU MEN SHIH CHING), said, "Only the learned know the truth, and those who attend the family should have medical knowledge."[17] This means that correct medical treatment should be based on a thorough theoretical and clinical education. It should not be based on half-truths or unproven assumptions. From the perspective of Chinese medicine, western allopathy and many so-called alternative therapies are lacking a complete picture of health and disease and are thus lop-sided. Although Zhang's work has been somewhat discredited, it is important to remember what of value he did put forward as well as what was wrong. It is only by reviewing the treasure of past experience recorded in the classics that modern practitioners of Chinese medicine can safeguard ourselves from deadends, false promises, and the futility of reinventing the wheel. And, in order to retain this ability to review the past, certain standards of scholarship and clear thinking must be maintained. Only thus can we, as "learned" persons, correctly minister to the needs of our family, the human race.

ENDNOTES

1 Kaptchuk, Ted J., THE WEB THAT HAS NO WEAVER, Congdon & Weed, NYC, 1983, p. 256-265

2 Chang Hsien-cheh, "The Concept of Pathology in Chinese Medicine after the Sung Dynasty", OHAI BULLETIN, LA, Vol. 9, #7, Nov. 1984, p. 334

3 Ibib. p. 334

4 Ibid. p. 336

5 Ingredients of ZHEN WU TANG:

Baked Aconite	9-12 grams
Atractylodes alba	10-15
Poria	10-15
Peony	6-9
Fresh Ginger	6-9

6 Smith, Reece & Dharmananda, Subhuti, "AIDS Prevention: Preliminary Considerations in the Management of the Prodrome symptoms Using the Concept(s) of Traditional Chinese Medicine", JACTCM, SF, #2, 1985, p. 20-29

Shanahan, Tom, "AIDS: Some Facts for the Acupuncturist", JCM, London, #18, May 1985, p. 11-18

Smith, Michael, "Acupuncture for AIDS", MEDECINE TRADITIONELLE CHINOISE ET ACUPUNCTURE, Quebec, Vol. 7, #7, July 1984, p. 25

7 Dubos, Rene, MIRAGE OF HEALTH, Harper & Row, NYC etc., 1979, p. 166

8 Ehret, Arnold, MUCUSLESS DIET HEALING SYSTEM, Dobbs Ferry, NY, 1983, p. 227

9 Walker, Norman W., COLON HEALTH: THE KEY TO VIBRANT LIFE, O'Sullivan, Woodside & Co., Phoenix, 1979, p. 11

10 Jensen, Bernard & Bell, Sylvia, TISSUE CLEANSING THROUGH BOWEL MANAGEMENT, Escondido, CA, 1981, p. 3

11 Ibid. p. 10

12 Burroughs, Stanley, THE MASTER CLEANSER, Auburn, CA, 1976, p. 1

[13] Tilden, J.H., TOXEMIA EXPLAINED, Keats Publishing, New Canaan, CT, 1981, p. 26

[14] Ibid. p. 47

[15] Jensen & Bell, op. cit., p. 4

[16] Ingredients in the Decoction for Warming the Spleen:

Rhubarb	6-9 grams
Aconite	6-9
Codonopsis	3-6
Dry Ginger	3-6
Licorice	3-6

[17] Chang, op. cit., p. 336

PLAYING THE BALL WHERE IT LIES

Descriminating BEN & BIAO in the Treatment of Hemoptysis

The descrimination between BEN (Root) and BIAO (Branch) is an important distinction in erecting a treatment plan according to Chinese medicine. This descrimination must be made based on the patient's immediate condition when seeing the practitioner and the practitioner's ability, using the physiologic theories of Chinese medicine, of prognosing the patient's condition in the future. Western practitioners beginning the study and practice of Chinese medicine often do not recognize that diagnosing why a symptom appeared in the past is not the same as diagnosing the patient in the immediate present. This tendency is, in my opinion, a function of two factors. First, most nephytes rely on textbooks to aid them in their diagnosis. Traditional Chinese medical textbooks typically will list the several most commonly encountered patterns of disharmony usually responsible for a given symptom or disease. The beginner who successfully is able to differentiate between such a list and identify their patient's etiology will feel as if their job is done and will also feel a certain sense of security that their patient matches the textbook description. This satisfies two common flaws of human nature: laziness and insecurity. Secondly, most westerners find it difficult to abandon the subtle but pervasive conditioning of the so-called modern, scientific medical model. This medical model emphasizes the naming of the disease as if it were a concrete entity. Although western practitioners of Traditional Chinese Medicine may criticize the pragmatic utility of a diagnosis that goes no further than describing a physical phenomenon, such as appendicitis, i.e. an inflammation of the appendix, still we often relate to Chinese energetic patterns of disharmony, such as Damp Heat or Stagnant Blood, as if they were entities in the same way.

The tendency to identify a patient's problem by giving it a name, even a Chinese energetic name, tends to freeze the image of the patient in time if the practitioner is not careful to the contrary. The essence of Chinese medicine is assessing the ebb and flow of Qi through the cycles of change which are an integral aspect of time. Inattentiveness to this quality of temporality and flux likewise leads to a less than artful employment of traditional Chinese therapeutics. It can often lead to errecting an erroneous treatment plan similar to closing the barn door after the horse has run away. That is not to say that we, as practitioners of Traditional Chinese Medicine, should abandon the use of the Differentiation of Syndromes (BIAN ZHENG). But, we should remember that such conceptualizations are only aids to help us relate to reality in a systematic and rational way. As such, categories such as Kidney Qi Deficiency and Spleen Dampness do not exist other than as partial descriptions of reality, i.e. as ideas. As practitioners of a medicine based on assessing and correcting the flow of Qi, we, perhaps more than other types of physicians, should guard ourselves from allowing the concepts we employ from freezing us from this nameless flow. As Lao-tze said, the five tones make us deaf.[1]

The following case history, I believe, exemplifies the importance of descriminating between BEN and BIAO. It also underscores the necessity of treating the present condition as opposed to an historical one. And it points out the necessity of understanding why a certain symptom arose when it did. Without that understanding, no prognosis can be made with any degree of probability. Dr. Shen of New York describes three levels of medical skill: "The first, the lowest, does not understand either the disease or the cause, but treats only the symptoms, and his results are not good. This is the level that much acupuncture in the West and nowadays in the East too is practised on. The second level doctor understands the condition, but not the cause and can often treat successfully, but the highest level understands the cause of disease in each patient."[2]

The patient was a twenty-five year old female. Eighteen months prior she had had an acute occurence of hemoptysis. For no apparent reason, she suddenly had begun to cough and brought up a Cup of fresh red blood. This happened three days in arow and then stopped. At that time, western medical examination could not find any cause for the hemoptysis and no treatment was given. Then, a year and a half later and three weeks before her visit to my clinic, she coughed up a handful of fresh red blood again. This time bronchioscopic examination revealed a pimple-sized lesion on her bronchi. The patient was advised to have surgery to remove this lesion. However, a second bronchioscope two weeks later showed no trace of this lesion and surgery was cancelled.

According to Chinese medicine there are four patterns of disharmony which may result in hemoptysis. They are: 1) Rebellious Qi, 2) Lung Yin Deficiency, 3) Toxic Heat in the Lungs, and 4) Stagnant Blood in the chest.[3]

Blood Stagnation hemoptysis is usually seen in patients over sixty with congestive Heart conditions. The blood that is coughed up tends to be dark and may be clotty. The patient's face is purplish red and dusky. Their lips and nail beds may be cyanotic. Usually they are fatigued, experience chest pain and Heart arrhythmia, and often they have dyspnea and edema in their lower extremities. Their tongue is dark red or purplish or may have purplish streaks or patches. Their pulse is usually deep, weak, and irregularly irregular (JIE MAI). Such patients will usually be under the care of a physician. They may be taking western allopathic medication for hypertension, arrhythmia, blood clots, edema, or cardiac asthma. In general this is a dangerously ill patient.

Toxic Heat (RE DU) in the Lungs is the energetic pattern which usually causes purulent pulmonary abscess. This patient has a systemic fever, a parched mouth, and tends to be constipated. There is foul-melling, pussy mucous mixed with the blood. The tongue fur is yellow and the pulse is rapid. Such a situation can be caused by repeated pulmonary infections or long periods of coughing with abundant sputum. It may also be caused by a foreign body lodging in the Lungs and decomposing. This could be caused by loss of consciousness with vomiting or post-oral surgery accompanied by ineffective material suction. The patient is likely to be weak, suffer from loss of appetite, and complain of chest pain and dyspnea. In other words, there is a history of Lung imbalance over some duration and the patient is visibly ill.

Lung Yin Deficiency likewise does not usually appear precipitously. Either the patient has suffered from Lung Fire which has severely scorched the Yin, in which case he or she would have had a fever and a sharp, painful cough for at least several days and probably have been sick in bed, or has a history of chronic Lung Kidney Yin Deficiency. In this case, the patient will have experienced a low-grade, chronic sore throat in the mornings and evenings or when fatigued. This may or may not be accompanied by a weak, shallow, dry cough. The patient may experience a low-grade fever or malar flushing in the afternoon or evening and/or may suffer from night sweats. Usually patients suffering from Lung Kidney Yin Deficiency tend to be thin. Hemoptysis may be caused in such cases by an acute pulmonary infection superimposed on top of a chronic Yin Deficiency or it may be caused by overwork, fatigue, stress, stimulants, drugs, or anything else which would substantially consume Yin. Such patients tend to appear fragile and somewhat nervous. Lung Yin Deficiency hemoptysis is typically seen in cases of pulmonary tuberculosis.

Rebellious Qi hemoptysis can be of sudden onset precipitated by stress. The tongue is normal. There is no phlegm, no preceding cold, flu, or pulmonary infection. The blood is bright red. And the pulse is wirey and slippery. The patient is otherwise in good health. This is the pattern of disharmony responsible for the present patient's hemoptysis. The patient's tongue was normal. Her pulse was slippery and a little bit wirey. It was not deep, weak, thready, fast, or irregular. She appeared extremely healthy but also appeared wirey like a high-spirited race horse. This type of purely functional hemoptysis which is unassociated with infection is very hard for western allopathic medicine to either diagnose or treat since allopathic medicine lacks the concepts which best describe its occurence.

According to A BAREFOOT DOCTOR'S MANUAL, Rebellious Qi hemoptysis can be treated by either acupuncture or herbs.[4] The suggested acupuncture treatment consists of needling CHI ZE (Lu 5), ZU SAN LI (St 36), LIE QUE (Lu 7), and YU JI (Lu 10). This, however, is a "shotgun" formula which does not adequately differentiate between the energetic etiologies of hemoptysis. Specifically for Rebellious Qi hemoptysis I would suggest needling SHAN ZHONG (CV 17), LIE QUE, HE GU (LI 4), ZU SAN LI, and YU JI (Lu 10). Since the patient did not have Lung Heat I would not have needled CHI ZE. SHAN ZHONG lowers rebellious Qi in the Upper JIAO. LIE QUE likewise lowers and regulates the Lung Qi and has a symptomatic effect on the throat and bronchi. Similarly, YU JI has a specific effect on the throat and bronchi and, although it is usually used for dispersing Heat, it also does lower Rebellious Qi.[5] HE GU and ZU SAN LI, important points regulating the YANG MING, control Rebellious Qi by indirectly strenghtening the Middle Qi and peristalsis, disperse Excess, and HE GU has a pronounced symptomatic effect on the throat as well. Furthermore, HE GU is the upper pair of the Four Gates and it therefore influences the regular flow of Qi kept patent by the dredging function of the Liver.

The suggested herbal formula given in A BAREFOOT DOCTOR'S MANUAL for Rebellious Qi hemoptysis consists of:

Raw Radix Rehmannia	15 grams
Radix Rubia	15
Cacumen biotae	12
Fructus Perillae	9
Radix Moutan	9

Raw Rehamnnia, Moutan, and Thuja (Cacumen Biotae) are all cooling to the Blood and arrest bleeding due to Heat in the Blood. Perilla seed lowers Rebellious Qi and Rubia is a hemostatic.

In any case, I did not choose to administer either of the above treatments. To do so would have been to treat a historical condition not currently present. Hemoptysis is a symptom, not a disease. It is an acute or Branch symptom. The treatment of acute symptoms is appropriate when they are currently manifesting. This is according to the principle of treating the BIAO in an acute case. Hemorrhaging is always seen as a BIAO symptom. "Bleeding (BIAO) must be stopped, no matter what the BEN."[6] However, at the time of seeing this patient, there had not been any bleeding for three weeks. According to the same author, "When bleeding stops, other methods are used to treat BEN."[7]

This last episode of hemoptysis had only occured one time and had not reoccured for one and a half years. This was hardly a continuously presenting symptom. Western bronchioscopy could find no trace of a current lesion. Therefore it was not likely that the patient was still on the verge of another episode. Other than the slippery pulse, there was no sign of Heat in the Blood or Rebellious Qi. And Rebellious Qi, in any case, is likewise not a complete diagnosis but only a description of an energetic aberration in the flow of Qi. As a concept it does not explain why the Qi is or was rebellious. So rather than treating the patient for Rebellious Qi hemoptysis, I sought deeper for a diagnosis of her BEN and for the cause of the episodic BIAO.

The patient described herself as being in perfect health. In reviewing her various physiologic functions, however, certain anomalies appeared surrounding her menstruation. Her period was a little long, a 30-35 day cycle. Her flow was scant and painless. However, premenstrually she suffered from emotional lability, tender and swollen breasts, a bloated lower abdomen, and cravings for sugar. These symptoms plus the slightly wirey quality in her pulse indicated Liver Qi Congestion. This, in turn, explained the Rebellious Qi and the Heat in the Blood. (Although this syndrome is called simply Rebellious Qi in A BAREFOOT DOCTOR'S MANUAL, it is accompanied by a certain amount of Heat in the Blood even though the name of this pattern does not allude to it.)

The Qi moves the Blood and also holds the Blood within its channels. In the case of hemoptysis, Qi rebelling upwards drafts with it the Blood. The Liver promotes the free flow and patency of the Qi in the body. If the Liver becomes disordered, Qi flow may become aberrant. When the Liver Qi becomes congested, it often transforms into Heat due to the principle of Similar Transformation. Since the Liver stores the Blood, this Heat in the Liver can be transferred to the Blood stored in it. The source of Heat in the Liver is the Premier Fire or MING MEN HUO. Premier Fire is the source of Righteous Heat of the Kidney Yang but also of the Liver, Gallbladder, Stomach, Pericardium, and Triple Heater. As we all know, Heat has a tendency to rise.

The major cause of Liver Qi Congestion is emotional stress. Therefore, in attempting to determine why this patient's Qi had rebelled up suddenly three weeks previously, I questioned her regarding stresses in her life and anything which might have caused an exacerbation of Heat. The patient reported she had been about to leave for Europe in a couple of days. The night before the hemoptysis, she had drunk a largish amount of alcohol, had eaten sushi, and had smoked marijuana. Travelling is inherently stressful, particularly to the Liver since the changes in time zones, seasons, and living patterns upsets the regular flow of Qi. The negative effects of travelling are particularly apparent in airline flight attendants, a number of whom I have as patients. This patient had already and recently travelled across the continent on her way to Europe. The patient also admitted that she had been feeling very excited and nervous about her trip. Alcohol can both aggravate Liver Qi Congestion and inflame the Blood. As far as the sushi is concerned, it may also have been a precipitating factor. Certain types of fish, such as tuna, mackerel, sardines, lobster, and shrimp, can cause or aggravate Hot Blood. And finally, the marijuana certainly contributed to the onset of this hemoptysis in a very interesting way.

Marijuana acts in the human body like a key in a lock. It releases a gate mechanism which liberates a large amount of MING MEN Fire to flow up through the core of the body to the brain. It is this energy which causes the "high" of psychedelics. Normally this energy is locked in the pelvis and is parcelled out to provide the Heat for the organism's metabolic processes. Marijuana, LSD, peyote, psilocybin, etc. allow this energy to rush unchecked towards the Heavens. This energy is also called Kundalini. Tibetan medicine also uses the concept of the Gate of Life. In Tibetan it is called TSAM-TSE. TSAM meansgate or boundary and TSE means life. When Dr. Yeshe Donden was asked by a group of American allopathic physicians where this TSAM-TSE is located anatomically, Dr. Donden repleied that it is in the region of the prostrate. This is also the location of the Muladhara Chakra, the seat of the Kundalini. This energy can be used for maintenance of metabolic processes, for transformation and regeneration of the individual, for procreation, and for recreation, not all without their negative consequences.

Given the fact that the patient was thin and tended to be hyperactive, she normally generated more Fire than Water in her system and had probably a tendency towards her Blood being a little heated for some time. This was coupled with her tendency to Liver Qi Congestion which likewise typically overheats the Blood over time. When this underlying scenario was combined with the stress of travelling, the alcohol, and the upsurge of MING MEN Fire liberated by the marijuana, this resulted in the sudden rebelling of the Qi and the bubbling over of the "boiling" Blood thus causing the hemoptysis.

Although this patient may have a continuing tendency for this rebellion to happen again given the right circumstances, if she consciously minimizes her level of stress, is conservative with her use of alcohol, and avoids marijuana and other psychedelics altogether, it is my opinion that she is not likely to experience hemoptysis again. Therefore I did not seek to treat the hemoptysis directly either with herbs or acupuncture. However, without endeavoring to pinpoint the contributing causes of the Rebellious Qi, the practitioner would otherwise be in a quandry whether to treat it or not as a yet imminent possibility.

Instead I explained my logic to her regarding the scenario that resulted in her episode of hemoptysis. I counselled her on the negative effects of stress and gave her a list of foods which would aggravate her Liver Qi Congestion and Hot Blood. This included alcohol, coffee, caffeine, drugs, preservatives, chemicals, pollutants, heavy red meats in overabundance, greasey, oily, fatty foods, spicey, pungent, "hot" foods, and overindulgence in chicken, shrimp, and fish such as trout. Lastly we discussed at length the mechanics of marijuana intoxication and its effects on the Kidneys, on Premier Fire in general, and on the SHEN or Spirit.

Since the patient was again planning to leave for Europe in a week, I prescribed XIAO YAO WAN in patent medicine form. She could not carry a bulky herb prescription with her due to baggagge limitations and the likelihood that a customs official would confiscate such a suspicious looking parcel. Likewise, while travelling she would not have the time nor the regularity to make and take an herbal formula in tea form. XIAO YAO WAN are convienient to carry and take and are packaged in an unsuspicious way. XIAO YAO WAN's ingredients include: Bupleurum, Tang Kuei, Peony, Poria, Atractylodes, Mint, Ginger, and treated Licorice. Bupleurum deobstructs the Liver. Tang Kuei and Peony relax the Liver and to a minor extent cool the Blood in that they are sedative through nourishing the Blood. Poria and Atractylodes tonify the Spleen Qi and promote the transformation and transportation (YUN HUA) of Water. By keeping the Spleen Qi strong, these two ingredients indirectly promote Blood production. A strong Spleen also tends to help keep the Liver in balance. And finally, well regulated Water metabolism ensures moist Blood which is less prone to overheating. Mint also deobstructs the Liver and is mildly cooling to the Yang Ming. This helps keep the MING MEN HUO of the Stomach from becoming Excessive. Ginger and Licorice support the circulation of Qi and Blood and support the Middle Burner Qi. In the best of all possible worlds, I would have preferred to have the patient take a modified version of XIAO YAO TANG in decoction. In which case I would have deleted the Bupleurum, Mint, and Ginger and added Moutan and Raw Rehmannia. Bupleurum and Mint tend to dry the Yin. This patient's Yin, although not clinically Deficient was not robust and needs protection. Moutan and Raw Rehmannia directly cool the Blood. My feeling at the time was that the patent pill form of XIAO YAO WAN would not overdredge and therefore exhaust the Yin.

Since it was not possible to administer such a custom-tailored formula, I needled SAN YIN JIAO (Sp 6), XUE HAI (Sp 10), TAI ZHONG (Liv 3), and HE GU (LI 4). This was to cool the Blood, tonify the Yin, and release and relax the Qi. The patient was suggested to take the XIAO YAO formula, either in unmodified pill form or as an individually tailored prescription, for from six months to a year, since in my experience it is very difficult to eradicate the deep-seated tendency in many western women to Liver Qi Congestion. Although her premenstrual symptoms will probably improve in from two to three periods, she will be likely to fall back into a similar pattern in the future if either stress or diet become imbalanced. It is important for the patient not to abandon the XIAO YAO formula prematurely but to continue taking it for a long time to consolidate its therapeutic results. Because of the particular conditions our society, environment, and lifestyle have created, XIAO YAO formula is, in my opinion, one of the single most important formulae in the treatment of western women.

In any case, if we as western practitioners of Traditional Chinese Medicine are to go beyond a cookbook approach to treatment, we will need to study and understand more about time in relation to the evolution of patterns of disharmony and in relation to erecting treatment plans. The BEN/BIAO dichotomy is one way TCM has traditionally related to temporality in treatment. Textbooks, by their nature, tend to present static pictures of seemingly concrete entities. Now that a number of good Traditional Chinese Medical textbooks are available in western languages, it is hoped that more case histories and the records of individual practitioners, both classical and contemporary, will also become available since it is only by studying these that a sense of the the living process of Chinese medicine is gained through reading.

Case History Update: Eight months since first writing this essay the above-mentioned patient returned to see me. She reported that she had not had any further recurrence of hemoptysis and that her PMS was very much improved. We discussed the possibility of XIAO YAO WAN causing Yin Deficiency complications but the patient reported that she had not experienced any and requested that she be allowed to continue taking these pills. The patient said she felt much calmer and not so "speedy" when she took these pills. Checking her pulse I found it to be still wirey but not slippery.

ENDNOTES

1 Lao-tze, TAO TE CHING, Chapter 12

2 Deadman, Peter, "Dr. Shen Seminar, London, August 1979", THE JOURNAL OF CHINESE MEDICINE, collected reprints from issues 1-6, London, p. 15

3 Revolutionary Health Committee of Hunan Province, A BAREFOOT DOCTOR'S MANUAL, Cloudburst Press, Mayne Isle & Seattle, 1977, p. 94

4 Ibid. p. 94

5 Mann, Felix, THE TREATMENT OF DISEASE BY ACUPUNCTURE, William Hienemann Medical Books Ltd., London, 1974, p. 5

6 Qiu Mao Lian & Su Xin Ming, THE NANJING SEMINAR TRANSCRIPT, transscribed & edited by Peter Deadman, The Journal of Chinese Medicine, London, 1985, p. 86

7 Ibid. p. 86

SEEING THE FOREST

A Case Study in Retained Placenta

Once, the enigmatic and well-known Michael Broffman asked a group of students to pair up and draw each other's face. He wanted to emphasize that the first job of the practitioner of Chinese medicine is to simply observe without prejudice and without interpretation. In looking, listening, palpating, and questioning, one should first collect the data before assigning a meaning to each individual sign and symptom. Only then, after having collected the raw information, should the practitioner go back and interpret this information. In doing so, he or she must attempt to account, in a logically consistent way and according to the theories of Chinese energetic physiology, for every peice of information. In other words, no piece of information should be discarded because it does not fit our hypothetical diagnosis. We may emphasize one set or series of data as being more relevant to the case at hand, as when one choses to emphasize the symptoms above the pulse or the pulse above the symptoms, but still we should endeavor to understand whatever apparent anomalies appear. Michael Broffman has always insisted on seeing the patient as they are, not as we might wish they were because that would be intellectually easier for us.

All too often neophytes seek security in assigning a single meaning to each single sign and symptom. For instance, a red-tipped tongue means Fire in the Heart. Often this sign does mean that, but it can also point to Liver Heat as well as Heat due to Stagnant Blood. Likewise, when feeling the pulse, beginners when queried about what they feel will often respond that they feel this or that organ is strong or weak. What they should report is only a description of the feeling of the pulse, whether it is weak, deep, soft, thready, etc. Whether an organ is weak or not because of feeling some quality in the pulse may or may not be accurate. The meaning of what one is feeling under their fingers is dependent upon the entire conformation of the case and not on any absolute system of tit-for-tat correspondences. One may, in feeling the CHIH position sunken, jump to the conclusion that the Kidney is weak. Although this does mean that the Righteous Qi in the Lower JIAO is not circulating at parr, immediately interpreting this as Kidney Deficiency is too simplistic. It may also be due to retardation of the Qi and Blood or to problems in the Intestines or Bladder or even in the legs. What it actually does mean in a particular patient depends on the total complex of signs and symptoms seen in relation to each other. I remember how frustrating it was as a beginner to ask Michael Broffman what this or that symptom meant and always being told that that depended on a number of variables, often chief of which was the relation in the time of onset of a given symptom to the other symptoms. At the time it seemed like I could never get a straight answer out of Michael. Now the response, "This is a large discussion", is remembered with rueful fondness.

Students beginning the study of Chinese medicine learn lists of correspondences. Unfortunately, when these are presented as lists, charts, and tables in modern texts, all too often there is not the cautionary explanation that these are only probabilities. Usually a certain sign means this. Most of the time a certain symptom means that. The learning of such lists is like learning the vocabulary of a foreign language. One must learn these lists before one can begin. But once one has learned them, the preceptive student will see that what is really required is the ability to think and reason according to the logic and language of Chinese medicine.

When dealing with a single problem in a previously unseen patient, it may be difficult for the beginning practitioner to capture the sense of a living, changing, evolving situation. The so-called Differentiation of Syndromes (BIAN ZHENG) approach to Traditional Chinese Medicine tends to reinforce the attitude that diseases and imbalances are discrete entities. In an attempt to identify a section of the continuum of physiologic and energetic imbalance, conceptual compartments have been created which masquerade as real things, which in actuality are only pragmatic descriptions in the Deweyan sense. However, when one sees a single patient over a period of years and watches them go through various permutations and progressions of their situation, one comes to appreciate Chinese medicine's ability to pragmatically conceptualize these changes in a consistent and rational way. One begins to see various patterns of disharmony not as separate diseases but as part of a flow which has its highs and lows, twists and turns, and meetings and partings, all of which are reasonably predictable if the practitioner has enough information and is able to think in terms of Chinese theory.

When treating women during pregnancy, the evolution of symptoms and patterns is very easy to see. On the one hand, pre and postnatal care is a good specialty in which to get a sense of the flowing quality of Chinese medicine. On the other, if one does not have this sense, one may provide erroneous treatment to patients whose situation, in terms of long-term repercussions and gravity, requires competent treatment. Pregnant women who are suffering from an imbalance of one sort or another will usually display certain symptoms or problems at various stages of their pregancy, labor, and peurperium. Being able to think in Chinese energetic terms, it is relatively easy to diagnose pregnant women based on their history. It is also relatively easy to project the evolution of an imbalance into the future and, by doing so, treat preventively. If instead, the practitioner sees each symptom or problem during pregnancy as a separate and unrelated problem, one is likely to misdiagnose and therefore mistreat the patient.

The following case history exemplifies how an insufficiently educated and experienced practitioner can misdiagnose and mistreat a patient because of 1) using an overly simplistic set of correspondences in a rigid way and 2) because of failing to see the continuous and evolving nature of the patient's disharmony.

The case began with a phone call at 9:30 AM one Sunday morning. A lay midwife who works in conjunction with an acupuncturist had delivered a baby of a twenty-two year old woman. Two hours later the placenta had still not been expelled. The acupuncturist was out of town and the midwife requested me to come and do acupuncture to help the woman expel the placenta. According to the midwife over the phone, the patient was exhausted after labor and it was her opinion that the placenta was retained due to Qi Deficiency. To corroborate that opinion she added that the patient's tongue was pale and white coated and that she had been taking SHIH ER and SHIH SAN TAI BAO WAN throughout her pregancy after a threatened abortion in the fifth month. Based on the midwife's information I packed some needles, a bottle of WU JIA SENG EXTRACT, and a box of EU YAN SANG BAK FOONG PILLS. It took me one hour to drive to the patient's home.

When I arrived, the patient was resting quietly in the birth bed. It was obvious that her Spirit was quite secure. The labor had been without complication and had lasted approximately six hours. It was her second birth. Her first child was two years old. There was no hemorrhaging and her blood pressure remained stable at 125 over 85. The newly born little girl was, based on skin sloughing and the size and shape of her feet, judged to be full term but weighed under five pounds. The midwife said the baby's Apgar was between 8 and 10. Upon examination, I found the patient's tongue meat was normally colored except for a red tip. The fur,however, was thick white. The patient's pulse had normal strength and size. It was neither deep nor superficial except in the CHIH position where it was bilaterally deep. Overall the patient's pulse was wirey and slippery with the simple wirey quality extending into the CHIH position. Based on these findings it did not appear to me to be a case of Qi Deficiency placental retention.

I asked the patient if she had had morning sickness with a bitter taste in her mouth, sour or acid eructations, and depression. She answered that she had. Also, as stated above, she had experienced considerable hemorrhaging during her fifth month. At that time the midwife had assumed that she had in fact miscarried because of the amount of blood discharged. Her acupuncturist had begun adminstration of SHIH ER TAI BAO WAN at this time to forestall the miscarriage. Soon after that, however, the patient developed cystitis. At this point her acupuncturist diagnosed this as Damp Heat and Kidney Deficiency based, according to the midwife, on the depth of the CHIH pulse. He prescribed ZHU LING TANG in granular extract for this condition. This had helped somewhat but had not completely eliminated the cystitis which had persisted right up until the birth. Then, based on assuming that the white fur and deep CHIH pulse indicated a Deficient Cold condition, the same acupuncturist prescribed BU ZHONG YI QI TANG, also in granular extract, during the last three weeks of gestation. The patient had taken this up until labor had begun. I also asked her about her periods prior to conceiving her first child and she told me she had had a history of incapacitating dysmenorrhea which was experienced on the first day of the flow. As the flow became more free flowing, the cramps diminished. And finally, I asked the patient about her bowel movements and found out that she had a tendency to sticky, soft stools.

Based on the patient's pulse, tongue, and history, my diagnosis was retention of placenta due to Liver Qi Congestion. I surmised that there might also be Stagnation of Blood as well. In addition but not affecting directly the expulsion of the afterbirth, the patient also suffered from Spleen Dampness. It was this Liver Qi Congestion which had caused the dysmenorrhea, morning sickness, threatened abortion, and depression and was now causing the retained placenta. The Dampness had probably developed during the morning sickness which had not been treated as it should have been. This Dampness dripping down from the Middle JIAO had caused the sticky, soft stools, and the cystitis.

The patient's acupuncturist had only needled ZHU BIN (Ki 9) twice during the pregnancy, at the end of the first and second trimesters, to presumably disperse Fetal Toxicity preventively in utero. If he had treated the patient for Muddy Stomach Qi and Liver Qi Congestion during the morning sickness, he would not only have provided relief from the nausea and depression for the patient immediately but would also have reduced the likelihood of the abruptio placentae with threatened abortion, the cystitis, and the present placental retention. Instead, the SHIH ER and SHIH SAN TAI BAO WAN had probably aggravated the Dampness due to their containing "greasey" ingredients. Also the tonification of a patient with an Excess congestion had probably exacerbated that congestion. My feeling was that the TAI BAO WAN had not prevented the miscarriage since the formula is based on the principle of tonification rather than on deobstruction. Therefore it should not have had a marked therapeutic effect on this particular pattern of disharmony. Likewise the ZHU LING TANG and BU ZHONG YI QI TANG were wide of the mark. ZHU LING TANG is primarily for simple Damp Heat in the Bladder. Although Polyporus, Alisma, and Poria were indicated, these needed to be appended to a Liver Qi deobstructing and Spleen invigorating formula for best result. BU ZHONG YI QI TANG raises the Central Qi and is usually used to keep things up, such as prolapsed stomach, uterus, anus, etc. It seems a strange and antithetical choice to tonifying formula during the last few weeks of pregnancy when one wants the energy to descend even if, as was not the case, the patient had in fact needed tonification. Further, this formula is not a Warming formula and is not indicated in Deficiency Cold even if that were also the case.

When doing obstetrical acupuncture, my procedure is to begin with minimal intervention and add subsequent intervention only as it becomes apparent that these are necessary. Therefore I began by inserting needles in SAN YIN JIAO (Sp 6) and HE GU (LI 4). This caused several contractions within three minutes of insertion but these contractions did not push the placenta any further out. Next I needled QI HAI (CV 6) and ZHONG JI (CV 3). The contractions continued and the patient experienced some lower abdominal cramping. From time to time the midwife gently tugged on the cord. Each time the patient felt a slight pain and tugging in her uterus indicating that, in fact, the placenta was not "hung up" on the cervix but was still at least partially attached to the wall of the uterus. After another twenty minutes of contractions and cramps but no placenta, nor even any vaginal discharge of blood, I decided that the problem at this point was not only Stagnation of Qi but definitely Stagnant Blood as well. Based on this, I moved the needle at QI HAI down to GUAN YUAN (CV 4) and added needles at DI JI (Sp 8). Again we waited but again there was no discharge of the placenta.

By now the patient felt the need to urinate. Therefore I withdrew all of the needles so she could go to the bathroom. When she returned to her bed I did not reinsert the needles but instead suggested the father go to a local healthfood store to purchase two or three packages of TOKAKUJOKITO marketed by the San Francisco Herb T Co. This is the Japanese version of TAO HO CHENG QI TANG. As marketed by this company, its ingredients are only one third the usual contemporary Chinese dosage. This is a very strong LI XUE formula. It is a Blood destagnator and a purgative. Its ingredients include: Semen Persica, Radix Rheum, Radix Glycyrrhiza, Cortex Cinnamon., and Mirabilitum.

It took the father well over an hour to find and return with these herbs. He also returned with two packets of TWO PEONY ROOT TEA (GUI ZHI FU LING TANG) which I had also asked him to buy. During his absence I had applied Ginger and Myrrh hot compresses to the patient's lower abdomen which relieved the cramping she was experiencing since the acupuncture. This cramping was caused by the stimulation of the Qi and Blood in the area which was running up against the Blood Stagnation. As soon as the father returned with the herbs I brewed up a double dose of the TAO HO CHENG QI TANG and had the patient drink two thirds of a Cup of it. After waiting fifteen minutes, I inserted needles at SAN YIN JIAO, XUE HAI (Sp 10), TAI CHONG (Liv 3), and GUI LAI (St 29), a protocol I often use for Stagnant Blood in the Lower JIAO causing problems in the female reproductive organs. After another fifteen minutes the patient felt something "slip over a lip" or "unhook" two times in fairly quick succession. We could also hear gas rumbling in her intestines. I checked the pulse and it had clearly lost a great deal of its wiriness. I announced that we were all almost finished with our various labors. I asked the patient if she needed to defecate and she said that she would like to urinate. I withdrew the needles and the patient went to the bathroom. While sitting on the toilet she passed the placenta with the aid of manipulations by the midwife.

Examination of the placenta confirmed that the baby was indeed full term. It also displayed necrotic areas where it had detached at five months. The baby's low birth weight was most likely due to this unhealthy placenta. The placenta was also covered with blood clots and dark purple blood.

After the expulsion of the placenta there was still no lochia. Therefore, before leaving, I suggested that the patient take one pack of the GUI ZHI FU LING TANG per day for two days in order to try to destagnate the Blood further and establish a healthy lochia. This formula is likewise a LI XUE formula but it is a less drastic purgative. Its ingredients include: Cortex Cinnamon, Radix Peony, Poria, Radix Moutan, and Semen Persica. After taking this for two days I advised her to get in touch with her acupuncturist to check her out and to continue promoting her post partum discharge in an appropriate way. I stressed that it was important that both she and he work on Qi and Blood vitalization and not tonification and also on her Spleen Dampness. Since it was Summer and since the patient's pulse and tongue did not suggest Deficiency, I felt that if her digestion were regulated and invigorated she would have no trouble recuperating from the pregnancy and labor. On the other hand, tonification at this point would only exacerbate the Qi and Blood Stagnation and would tend to set in motion a trend which would result in the growth of pelvic neoplasms. Hopefully her acupuncturist was able to both hear this advice and implement it successfully.

This case had a relatively happy ending. Whether the patient's acupuncturist and midwife were able to correctly manage her post partum discharge is not known to me. Because the placenta is the baby's tissue and because it was so clotty and necrotic, I wonder if the child already does not have Congenital Stagnant Blood. If at menarche she, like her mother, suffers from dysmenorrhea, it should be inferred that this is due in part to her mother's pregnancy being less than artfully managed.

Until as practitioners we understand why symptoms and signs appear as they do and until we can see named patterns of disharmony as only sections of a continuing flow, western practitioners will continue to apply Chinese medicine from a symptomatic and overly simplistic point of view. Some westerners may blame the relatively scant amount of translated material available on the clinical practice of Chinese medicine as their main impediment to more skillful practice. But the beauty of the Chinese system is that because of its logical consistency, one can reason out with a fair degree of probability what has not been learned specifically from a book, lectures, or supervised clinical experience. However, for this to be possible we must be willing to do two things. The first is to think both rigorously and deeply. The second is to avoid projecting what we think we know onto situations inappropriately because this leads us to a safe, i.e. already known, conclusion. We must be willing to stick with our experience of our patients as they present themselves and avoid projecting onto them our intellectual timidity.

GIVING THE DRAGON EYES

A Discussion of the Merits of Apprenticeship In Chinese Medical Training

Several years ago, of several hundred practitioners who sat for the California acupuncture licensure examination, not a single American passed whose training consisted solely of apprenticeship. This led many in that state to proclaim that this method of acupuncture education is inefficient and out-dated. In the last ten years, more than fifteen "colleges" of Acupuncture have been established in America. Their course of study usually runs from two to four years maximum. Many of these schools require for admission college-level, western science pre-requisites, such as chemistry and physics. In fact, there is a movement afoot to eventually upgrade the entrance requirements to American acupuncture schools to the equivalent of a standard pre-med bachelor's degree. A national commission exists for the accreditation and standardization of these schools' curricula. The curricula at the majority of accredited American acupuncture schools have been patterned after similar, state-sponsored schools in the People's Republic of China. The American College of Traditional Chinese Medicine is widely regarded as the preeminent acupuncture school in the nation and most consciously patterns its approach to Chinese medicine and acupuncture after the theories and techniques taught at the Guangzhou, Shanghai, Nanjing, and Beijing Colleges of Traditional Chinese Medicine.

However, until this century and for at least two thousand years, the majority of Chinese acupuncturists and herbalists did not receive their education in schools with classes, graduation ceremonies, and diplomas but rather by apprenticeship. [1] The creation of contemporary colleges of Traditional Chinese Medicine was largely influenced by nineteenth and twentieth century ideas on science and education. Recognizing the efficiency of the western university for training large numbers of professionals, the Chinese adopted this system. This model of education was developed in the West to teach the materialist sciences which arose in the post-Renaissance period. Such a model, however, does not necessarily meet the organic needs of teaching Chinese medicine which is not such a materialist science. In fact, it seems to me that Chinese medicine has undergone a mutation so that it can be taught according to this educational model. Contemporary, so-called Traditional Chinese Medicine has adopted much of the methodology and criteria for determining value of western materialist science. Many, both easterners and westerners, who believe that the western scientific model of reality is the best and really real one, applaud this "demystification" and "scientification" of Chinese medicine. They see this streamlining as a positive step if Chinese medicine is to compete in the real, i.e. scientific, world of the late twentieth century. Yet others, such as myself, view this trend with serious misgivings.[2] Although I hardly believe anything just because it is antique or Oriental, I also know from personal experience that the type of Chinese medicine I believe is most capable of balancing the health needs of our time cannot be taught in group classes in a college curriculum.

Chinese medicine as taught by books and lectures and tested by multiple choice examination is, by necessity, linear. It assumes a straight forward deductive logic based on the accumulation of "facts". From this point of view, if one has memorized the relevant facts and has been taught to arrange these according to the logical process of Chinese medicine, one will be able to erect the "correct" treatment plan[3] which will rectify the patient's imbalance. This assumes a technical simplicity characteristic of western medicine which believes that if one correctly identifies the pathogenic bacteria and gives the antibiotic that kills this bacteria the patient will get well. However, as many patients of allopathy know, the restoration of health is not that easy as witnessed by the many infections treated by antibiotics which become chronic and recalcitrant.[4]

It is my experience that a number of non-linear factors play a part in the healing process. Although I believe that the logic of contemporary TCM is a superior one to, for instance, allopathy, I also do not believe it is totally complete or adequate. Just as a map is not identical to the terrain it represents, in the same way TCM diagnoses are only pragmatic abstractions. In particular I do not think that modern TCM theory and practice take into adequate account the energy of the physician, both physical and spiritual, as a significant factor in the healing process. Nor does it pay adequate attention to time and place both in arriving at a diagnosis and in erecting a treatment plan. As practiced in China today, it does not pay adequate attention to preventive care over years and decades nor does it do justice to the philosophical and spiritual concepts inherent in its conceptual matrix. It tends to emphasize the technical employment of professionally administered therapies, such as acupuncture, and does not take full advantage of exercise, meditation, diet, and other self-administered regimes which traditionally Chinese culture and medicine have developed to a high level. It has become increasingly compartmentalized so that patients either are treated by acupuncture, herbs, or massage but rarely by a multimodal approach using all of these in a carefully delineated and orchestrated treatment plan. In part this last shortcoming is based on the requirement of training a technician in less than five years and therefore only being able to train a person in one limited modality. The main fallacy of this approach to training and practice, as I see it, is its assumption that anyone, given the proper facts and procedures, can and should be a healer.

The healing encounter between patient and practitioner is an interpersonal relationship. It is not a cut and dry, objective situation. It is by nature subjective. This is especially so in Chinese medicine where symptoms, i.e. subjective reports by the patient, are often more important than signs or "objective" observations by the practitioner. In western medicine where these signs are increasingly the product of quantitative measurements, there is the illusion of objectivity, as long as we discount the fact that all data are registered in the mind of the beholder. In Chinese medicine, where these signs are exclusively based on the practitioner's sense of sight, touch, hearing, and smell, even these signs are, by nature, subjective to the practitioners. The traditional apprenticeship training of the Chinese or Oriental doctor is based on the subjective nature of its data and process. Therefore such training is not confined to the memorization of information and the perfection of technical skills. Rather it includes the training and development of the entire person on physical, energetic, mental, emotional, and spiritual levels designed to create a healer. The development of the potential practitioner's sensitivity, physical energy, mental clarity, moral fiber, intuition, compassion, and spiritual power are all integral aspects of this training and, in fact, these are typically given precedence over technical knowledge or skill. Even regarding intellectual knowledge and technical skill, the level of proficiency is usually much higher in practitioners trained in this way. This difference in proficiency is especially evident amongst American practitioners since the entire methodology of our education and culture tends to foster superficiality.

In Asia there are consciously employed, systematic trainings for developing the mind, Heart, body, and Spirit. Such trainings have evolved over several thousands of years and scores of generations. These trainings were developed by individuals and groups who devoted their entire lives to the understanding of the principles and mechanisms of human growth. Often these individuals spent their entire lives in seclusion, on mountaintops, in monasteries, and in caves, where they experimented on themselves within the laboratory of their own organism with a single-mindedness hard for contemporary westerners to even imagine.[5] In China these explorers of human potential were most often Buddhist and Taoist monks but were also often devout Confuscianists.[6] Although we tend to think of Confuscianism as a social and moral philosophy, many of its adherents practiced self-cultivation with religious fervor equal to the saints of any religious tradition. Since the Ming dynasty, this type of training of the entire individual has also been promulgated by marital artists of many lineages. In fact, the words KUNG FU simply mean accomplishment through discipline. Therefore a KUNG FU adept is not necessarily or primarily a fighter.

Such trainings of the body, mind, and Spirit are rigorous and require great perseverance. Not everyone who attempts them succeeds. Since these trainings usually create supranormal power and abilities, teachers have to be absolutely sure of the moral character of the student. Therefore an essential part of such training is testing and commitment. Certain character traits have been traditionally and pragmatically recognized as being necessary checks and balances within such a trained individual. Ways to develop missing or weak character traits have been developed over generations.

Since every potential practitioner is an individual with idiosyncratic character, talents, and abilities, there can be no hard and fast, standard form to one's shaping as a healer. The apprenticeship of one traditional student may look very different from another student's even under the same master. When I asked Huang Pao-chin, a traditionally trained doctor and KUNG FU man from Taiwan, what commitments are generally required by traditional teachers, he replied that usually the teacher will watch and test the potential disciple for several

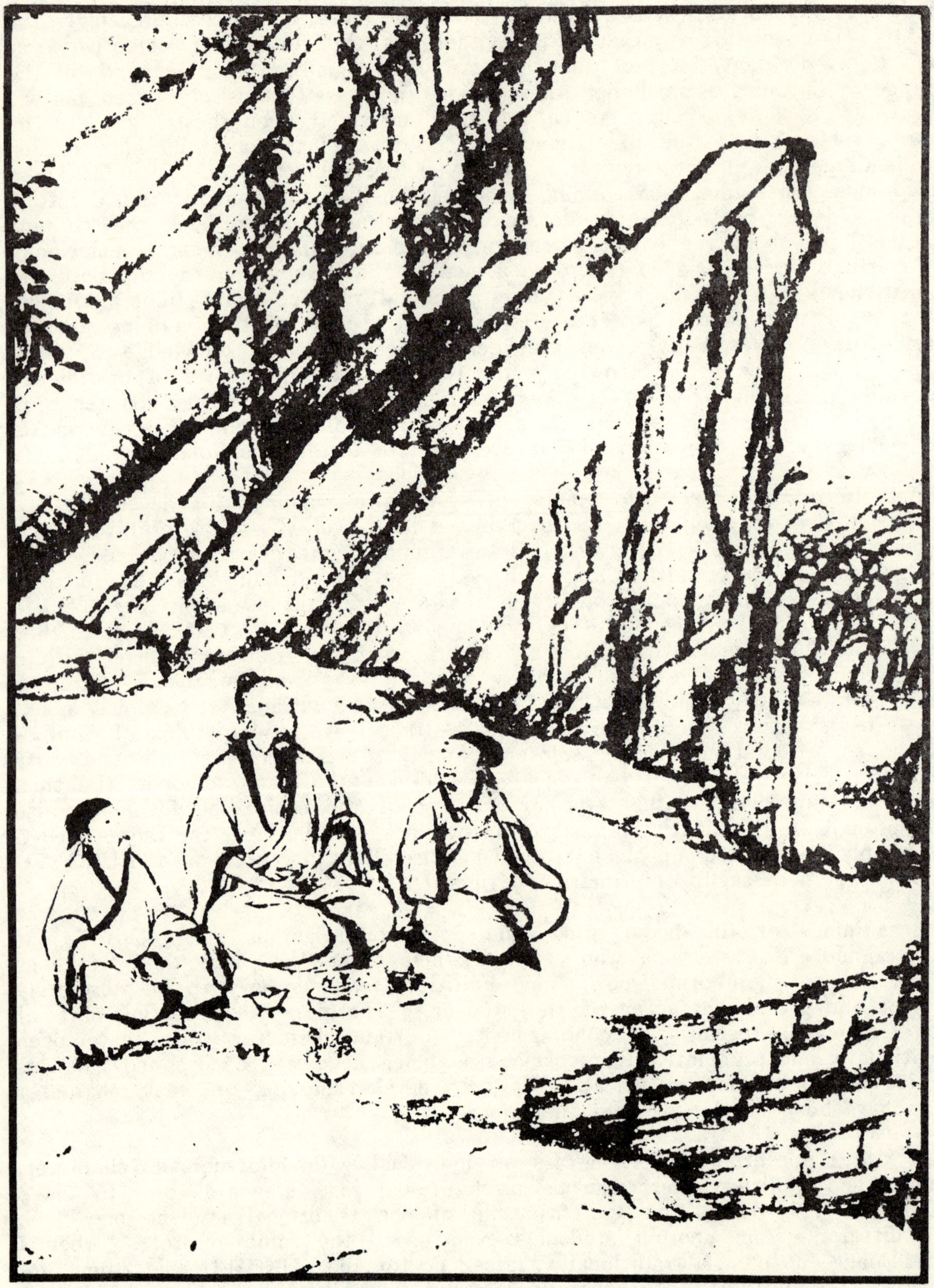

years. The specific commitments the student is finally required to abide by, even vow to, depend upon the needs of the individual student. However, most traditional apprenticeships are based on the development of patience since it is only patience and forebearance which allow the subsequent development of profundity and integrity.

My first acupuncture teacher, Dr. Tao Hsi-yu, began his study of the art under the tutelage of his uncle in his family tradition. Every day he had to empty and clean the honeypot and slops pail, sweep the house, run errands, and wait on his teacher. Often a month or more would go by without his uncle even mentioning acupuncture to him. These tasks and duties were meant to test his character, his perseverance, and his humility. Later on his uncle would teach him one new acupuncture point per day. To this day Dr. Tao can recite all three hundred sixty points on the fourteen meridians in order beginning with the Hand TAI YIN. A Chinese herbalist acquaintance likewise learned his art in his family's tradition. Whenever he did something meritorious in school or at home, his father or grandfather would reward him with a MI FANG or '"secret" formula from the family repertoire. Donn Hayes, a Colorado practitioner of Chinese medicine, underwent such an apprenticehsip with Huang Shu-li. For months he was asked to sweep the floors and clean the clinic without even any discussion of acupuncture. One day, he noticed that the characteristic change in the patient's energy due to treatment happened before the needles were inserted. He mentioned this observation to his teacher. His teacher beamed and said, "Now we can begin."

Ge Hung states in no uncertain terms the development of character based on patience and perseverance universally believed by all traditional Oriental teachers to be the basis of all accomplishment:

> Not a single of them (successful masters) failed to carry his package of books and resort to a teacher to perform many acts of labor. They underwent frost and dangers and were combed by the wind and bathed by the rain, as they personally did the sprinkling and sweeping and worked away in the art in widely separated places. They revealed themselves first in acts of faith, and in the end they were tried by perils and hardships.[7]

Ge Hung goes on to say:

> If found to be sincere and steadfast, their hearts and minds free from rancor and doubts, they were allowed to ascend into the hall and enter the home of their masters. Some grew weary and stopped in midcourse; others withdrew out of resentment and dissatisfaction. Some, enticed by worldly glory and advantages, returned to engage in lay pursuits; others won over by perverse arguments, lost their will to tranquility. Some became active in the morning and wished their task completed in the evening: others worked at their ease and expected immediate reults. It would be an overstatement to claim that there is even one man in ten thousand whose heart and mind are unmoved by the sight of wealth or beauty, and whose will is not weakened by the talk of the common herd.[8]

In terms of this training in character, all traditional Oriental life-arts value and stress the importance of patience and perseverance. It is assumed that the Superior Man can accomplish or master all things but that the inferior person can master nothing since he has not first mastered himself. Huang Pao-chin, in discussing this point, mentioned that if one masters one Chinese science or art, one has mastered them all. This is because it is assumed that a certain change in the character and personhood of the individual has taken place in the process of mastery which allows one access to the foundations of all knowledge and the principles of all phenomena.

There is a story of a Japanese samurai who, recognizing the precarious and ephemeral nature of his existence due to his duty, came to terms first with his mortality. Later he decided that he should also study fencing. When he went to a famous swordsmaster, the teacher looked at him long and hard. He asked the prospective student with whom he had studied and the samurai told the teacher he had not previously studied the sword. The teacher said that this was impossible since his eye told him this man was a master. The samurai replied that the only thing he had mastered was his fear of death. At that the teacher replied that he had tried to teach many students before the essence of swordsmanship but none had learned. But now he was sure that this samurai would learn in no time. He made the man his lineal successor on the spot. Similarly, Chogyam Trungpa, a Tibetan Lama, whose mind and character have been trained since he was five years old, is, in addition to being a Spiritual Teacher, an accomplished calligrapher, poet, landscape artist, and flower arranger. These accomplishments are not the result of lengthy training or apprenticeship in each but are a natural expression of his mastery of life. Likewise, my Teacher can seemingly do everything: paint, sculpt, garden, sing, dance, play numerous instruments, speak several languages, etc., because he has mastered the doing of nothing. Even in my own limited experience, I was able to learn Rolling Technique TUI NA from Dr. Ting Ji-feng very quickly for two reasons. The first was becuase I was able to listen to him and be open to his transmission. This in turn was due to my having undergone discipleship with other teachers. The second was because, having practiced the martial arts where repeating a punch or kick literally thousands of times a day is a common practice, I had already recognized the value of such repetitive and relatively boring practice. In addition, this previous physical training developed my kinetic skill and sensitivity which are the basis of any manual art.

Below are the general vows adhered to by members of the Buddhist medical lineage to which I belong. They are offered as an example of the commitments and ethics of one traditional Oriental medical lineage. These are found in the SHAY-GYUD, the second volume of the GYUD-ZHI, the Tibetan medical canon.

The eleven vows a doctor must take are:

(1) A person undergoing medical training must have great regard for his Teacher, considering him like a God.

(2) He must believe in whatever his Teacher teaches him and have no doubt whatsoever in his teachings

(3) He must have great respect for the books on medicine

(4) He must keep good, friendly relations with classmates, having regard and respect for each other.

(5) He must have sympathy towards patients.

(6) He should not regard the secretions of patients as filth.

(7) He must regard the Medicine Buddha and other medical experts as the guardians of medicine.

(8) He must regard medical instruments as holy objects and keep them properly.

(9) He must regard medicine as something very precious, something that fulfills all wishes.

(10) He must regard medicine as a deathless nectar.

(11) He must regard medicine as an offering to the Medicine Buddha and all the other medicine dieties.[9]

From a western materialist point of view these vows may seem superstitious. The meaning of the first vow is that the student should regard the teacher as the emanation of the Medicine Buddha. He should think that whatever the teacher does, says, or thinks is a teaching for the student. In other words, the student is asked to look into his own experience and see the coincident appropriateness of his relationship with the teacher. This goes deeper than a simplistic literal acceptance. When practiced correctly, this first vow creates great power and profundity in the student. The second vow means that the student's first job is to listen and contemplate deeply the teachings he receives instead of immediately arguing or concocting his own version. Deep teachings require time to mature and be understood. Respect in this tradition is not just a matter of mental respect. Therefore the third vow means that the student should show physical and verbal respect to the medical classics and not just intellectually value them. This means they should not be put on the floor, on a chair, walked over, used to rest something else on, leaned on, etc. This physical respect engenders a mindfulness which helps sharpen the intellect and instils a sense of importance of medical knowledge and practice deep in the core of the practitioner. The fourth vow means that the practitioner must develop compassion towards all patients without regard to friend or foe, rich or poor, attractice or ugly, etc. In Buddhist medicine there are a large number of spiritual practices which develop sympathy, compassion, joy at the well-being of others, and equanimity towards all in a step-by-step, systematic way. Vows eight through eleven all have to do with developing mindfulness and value. They invest all aspects of the practice of healing with the power of single-mindedness. They create a charged atmosphere in which the healer is the servant of the Infinite.

In my experience, if one has successfully gone through such a training with one teacher, other traditional teachers will recognize this fact. They will then accept the student readily without requiring much additional testing. They will share both their knowledge and techniques without coyness or hesitation and will transmit their power to the student. Such teachers recognize the qualities of the student through their body language, facial expression, choice of words and general deportment. Therefore, two students may approach a single teacher and one may study with that teacher a relatively short time and be given or receive a great deal, while the other student may study for years and years and hardly come away with anything. Since most Americans have not undergone such trainings and successfully completed them with one teacher (not that there is any real completion to such a relationship), most Americans have difficulty studying with traditional Oriental teachers. In many cases, American students don't even know that they are being tested and therefore don't recognize the need for patience, perseverance, and humility. I have heard one director of an American acupuncture school say that, by and large, Orientals are poor teachers, that most American teachers are able to put out more information more clearly in a shorter period of time. This totally misses the point of the traditional Oriental educational approach which is not based on the transmission of information alone or even primarily. Another well-known American practitioner of Chinese medicine who studied in China refused to "play the game" the way the Chinese do. Although he lived there for several years, he was never able to modify his appearance and demeanor to meet the Chinese expectations and therefore he remained an outsider. This man experienced a great many frustrations and problems during his study in China and came away with the view that the Chinese are not very nice. However, those Americans who have been able to modify their behavior to meet Oriental standards of studentship have had a very different experience of their teachers and have received a very different education.

It is also widely believed in Asia that hearing a teaching from a flesh and blood teacher is qualitatively different from merely reading it from a book. This is an aspect of discipleship commonly overlooked by most western critics. However, it is without doubt my experience that such is the case. I rarely really grasp something until it has been explained to me by a living teacher no matter how much I have read about the subject. The teacher may only repeat what the student has or will read but the living transmission creates a definite and special effect within the student. In the Buddhist lineage to which I belong this belief is so strong that no practitioner would think of picking up a scriptural text and reading it for practical purposes without receiving it orally from a living teacher who in turn received it in an unbroken lineage from its originator. As a corollary of this, it is also believed that one can only elicit in another the level of understanding they themselves have actually attained in a given subject. Therefore Asians often spend considerable time and effort to gain specific teachings from specific teachers. Even if an old master may speak imperfect English or speak with the idiosyncracies of age, it is believed that the depth of their understanding will shine through the limitations of their outward presentation and plant a special seed in the heart and mind of their student. Such certainly is my experience with both my spiritual Masters and several of my Chinese medical teachers.

The practice of all medicine is based on judgement. Chinese medicine is based on a particular logic with which its judgements are arrived at. It is a systematic way of thinking. One's ability to think within this system is therefore dependent on one's ability to think in general. Clarity is the criterion for successful thought and there are ways of developing mental clarity. Such methods are normally a part of most traditional Oriental apprenticeships. Memorization is one such technique. Chinese medical classics are terse and epigrammatic. Their logic is rigorous and spartan. Traditional students are often required to memorize entire books line for line. To fascilitate this, many mnemonic devices are used and many classics are written in meter and verse with rhyme. When a student makes a judgement, they are often required by their teacher to substantiate that judgement by quoting chapter and verse from a relevant classic. This instils the logic of the classic in the mind of the practitioner. It sharpens attention to detail. It develops presence of mind and it develops memory. In my tradition, a great deal of the transmission of information is done orally. Students are required to remember the words used, their meaning, and their order of presentation. As a saying goes in our tradition, even if chased by a pack of dogs, one should know their lessons so well that they could recite them flawlessly while running down the street. It is true that information can be looked up as needed but there are positive benefits to memorization besides the retention of facts. Leon Chaitow fails to appreciate this aspect of traditional training entirely when he writes: "Some people argue that before using acupuncture the practitioner should memorize all the points on the surface of the body ... The memorization of all the points on the body is not necessary for the successful application of acupuncture techniques ... points can be looked up as and when needed."[10]

The benefits of this method of training the mind are generally lost on westerners whose educational system has abandoned memorization, prefering to rely on an external data bank to recall facts and figures. In general, our system has abandoned its traditional methods for training intelligence and clarity of thought (Latin, Greek, grammar, geometry, etc.) and most young Americans consider logic and rationality perjorative terms. Since we can hardly think rationally in terms of our own language and culture, we have even greater difficulty understanding the logic embodied in a different culture and language. Recently, a student remarked to me that she was having difficulty learning Tibetan grammar since she had never learned English grammar. Chinese medicine is a very sophisticated conceptual system which is one of the flourescences of Chinese culture. It is not a conceptually simple system and simple and untrained minds have difficulty mastering it. In my experience, the best Chinese doctors are highly educated persons in all aspects of their culture. In addition to being physicians, they are also often calligraphers, poets, painters, geomancers, philosophers, and savants. As stated in a recent issue of THE PACIFIC JOURNAL OF ORIENTAL MEDICINE: "Healing is a philosophy, painting is a philosophy, and in China philosophy is one."[11] In the medical museum of the Shanghai College of Traditional Chinese Medicine there is a collection of Qing dynasty prescriptions written in calligraphy. I once received a similarly calligraphed prescription from an eighty year old Chinese doctor in Toronto who used all three syllable names for the ingredients to balance the formula visually and orally. On the facing page is likewise an example of a Chinese doctor's calligraphic composition of his medical theories and experience. These exemplify a refinement of sensitivity and a clarity of thought rarely encountered in modern medical circles. Such attention to detail and finesse of necessity require composure and consideration. One dose of the old Toronto doctor's prescription administered in his office immediately relieved the symptoms of a problem several weeks of other herbal formulae had failed to correct.

Over several thousands of years Asians have developed other methods for training mental clarity and memory. These include meditative techniques. In my own tradition, the visualization and mantric meditation on Manjusri, the Bodhisattva

右以内傷虚損而天分損之何可不立一膏滋之方方名助仙丹

白术 三錢 白芍 三錢 山藥 三錢 茹 一錢 杜仲 一錢

遠志 五分 陳皮 五分 炙甘草 二分

水煎服此劑宜仍如其舊不可每服也此方補中有

妙理健脾益胃解鬱清痰不損其天然之氣血使

中醫

黃仲衡

先生
女士

白茯神 [illegible]

炒豬苓 [illegible]

[illegible]

[illegible]

清水四碗煎至一碗八分温服

85年5月26日　診所

[illegible]

再診攜回原方

of Wisdom, develops both the intelligence and the memory. This can not be explained rationally. It is a suprarational experience, however verifiable by anyone willing to undergo the training. No one can explain how a fact or memory arises in the consciousness. It just appears. We use the verb to think as if thinking were a process like changing a tire on a car. Thinking is by nature a mystical occurence and mystical means can manifest thoughts spontaneously in the mind. Therefore one can have access to knowledge not gained in the ordinary way. In the same way, visualization and mantric meditation on Bhaishajyaguru, the Medicine Buddha, develops intuitive insights into medicine and healing hard to explain to the uninitiated. This practice also develops other powers germane to healing.

Manfred Porkert in an essay entitled "The Intellectual Social Impulses Behind the Evolution of Traditional Chinese Medicine" describes the special mode of thought used in the practice of Chinese medicine. "What is true of Chinese thought in general holds equally true for its practical applications in Chinese medicine: It is primarily interested in function as opposed to substance. The cognitive mode leading to the systematic perception of functions is called inductive and synthetic; the cognitive mode by which substratums are perceived rationally is called causal and analytical. The scientist who uses the inductive and synthetic mode of cognizance will observe first, and then speculate on his observations; the scientist who applies the causal and analytic mode will first speculate and act, and after that he will observe. The analytic and causal exploration of substratums requires that active effort precede receptive cognition. The synthetic and inductive perception of functions calls for no initial action, but requires the observer to consciously suspend any activity that would interfere with the functions to be observed."[12] This is a very succinct description of the practice of many Oriental methods of formless meditation. It is no wonder then that practice of such formless meditation forms the basis of certain lineages' training in Oriental medicine. It also follows that Buddhist and Taoist adepts who typically practice such meditation would be well suited to employ the inductive methodology Porkert describes as the basis of the Chinese medical epistemological approach and as Porkert remarks, historically this has proven true.

It is my and many traditional cultures' belief that the healing encounter in part depends on a transfer of energy or power to the patient. This energy may come from the personal reservoir of Qi accumulated within the practitioner or it can be channeled from a higher source through the practitioner. Huang Pao-chin, in discussing the relative practice of acupuncture and TUI NA, has said that the practitioner of TUI NA has to have more QI than the acupuncturist. He then described herbal methods of tonifying the practitoner's Qi in order to more effectively administer TUI NA. While studying in Shanghai, one of my clinical preceptors was an adept at NEI KUNG TUI NA or Internal Energy Massage. He could rub one side of the torso and the heat could be felt all the way on the opposite side which would, in fact, become erythematous. He had practiced NEI KUNG every day for twenty years in order to develop and train this ability.

However, one can only accumulate just so much energy within themself and this energy can be depleted or exhausted. Therefore channeling energy from a higher source is another approach which is ultimately less deleterious to the practitioner. The Medicine Buddha meditation mentioned above is one such way of both accumulating healing energy within oneself and of channeling it through one. The energy of life, like any other energy, tends to flow from where it is concentrated to where it is scarce. This transfer may be accomplished through touch as in massage, acupuncture, and palm healing, or through empowered objects or medicine, or through thoughts, words, and physical presence. Often this ability to transfer energy to the patient is the single most important part of the healing encounter. One acupuncturist I know believes he is a channel of divine healing grace. He uses all AH-SHI points without diagnosis and he has a very high success rate.

Compassion is one aspect of the healing power of life. According to Buddhism, compassion is an integral characteristic of ultimate reality. Therefore the development of a healer's compassion is likewise a power which Buddhist doctors believe plays a large part in the effecting of a cure. Dr. Trogawa Rinpoche has said that the true compassion of the doctor alone can do much to alleviate an ailment even without medicine. In Tibet there is a story about Atisha Dipankara, a famous eleventh century saint, who one day had a headache. When his students asked him if he required medicine, he said that placing his head in the lap of his student Dromton would be sufficient since Dromton had really developed true compassion. In Buddhism and Buddhist medicine there is a whole series of exercises designed to step-by-step develop the attitude and power of compassion. Sun Si-miao believed this Buddhist training of compassion should be an integral part of every Chinese doctor's training and in some lineages it is. Sun Si-miao wrote: "To be a good physician, it will not suffice to be versed in Confuscian and Taoist literature. No one who has not read Buddhist books will experience love, compassion, and the joy of renunciation. One will not know when approaching patients how to form the vow to convey succour to all sentient beings in all their sufferings, without distinction of rank, fortune, age, beauty, friendship or intimacy, nationality, or intelligence. One will not succeed in considering all patients with evenmindedness, as one's most dear friends."[13]

Terry Clifford, in writing about Tibetan medicine, emphasizes this view common to many traditional Oriental medical lineages that the healer's state of mind is of utmost importance in the healing encounter: "All this points to the fact that Tibetan medicine strongly emphasizes the state of mind of the healer as a major part of the healing process. In the Tibetan view, the healer's state of mind is not just a moral question which has no effect on the patient. It is held to be a vitally important influence on his condition. The ability to effect spiritual cures depends on the healer's consciousness -- his meditative powers of concentration and the purity of his intention. Therefore whatever kind of medicine is being practiced, the Tibetan healer will also be practicing internally various mystic healing exercises, visualizations, mantras, etc."[14]

Another component of the healer's mental state vis a vis their ability to treat is their confidence. Doubt is a great maggot. It underminds the unity of one's being and action. If one undergoes certain tests and rigors to be finally accepted into an authentic lineage stretching back through time and including many great doctors or healers, this gives one further authority to practice. If such and such a great doctor tested and picked his successor who tested and picked his and so on down to me, then there is the sense of belonging similar to being picked as the successor of that original great healer. For instance, my own lineage stretches back to the great Indian doctor Jivaka, Lord Buddha's own physician. This is not just a source of pride in a negative sense but also a confirmation of my own appropriateness as a healer. Belonging to such a lineage gives me confidence and inspiration even if one discounts the traditional belief that actual healing energy is passed down through such lineages. Micheal Broffman once said that without being a member of such an authentic lineage it is very difficult to be a really successful healer.

On a more prosaic level, many of the training methodologies adopted by traditional preceptors are designed to develop especially acute sensitivities or skills. Micheal Broffman has described a number of these he underwent as a student in Taiwan. Michael studied primarily under Dr. Li Su-huai. However, Dr. Li sent Micheal to a number of other masters for specific aspects of his education. One was a blind masseur. While studying with this man, every day on entering his house, he would have to blindfold himself for the entire day. He not only learned massage as a blind student would, but also had to navigate the house, get his meals, and carry out the requests of his teacher, all blindfolded. This was to develop sensitivity of touch, hearing, and smell, and also to de-emphasize his dependence on sight. The herbalist to whom he was sent would present him with an herb without telling him its name or anything about it. He was given several days to eat, smell, touch, test, and try to discover the nature and uses of this herb. Only after reporting his experiences to his teacher would the teacher then bring out the books and discuss the herb intellectually. Huang Pao-chin likewise does not value intellectual learning alone. He has described with noticeable disdain herbalists who know their ingredients only through books. Rather instead he values those practitioners, even without degrees, who have grown up with the herbs since childhood in their families' pharmacies.

Dr. Li required Michael to experience various diseases in his own body.[15] He was given one month to create an internal environment conducive to an imbalance and to induce it, one month to hang out with the disease and its symptoms becoming familiar firsthand with them, and one month to treat and cure himself by the methods he had been studying. Micheal experienced in this way cholera, neurasthenia, and several other diseases. Not only was this to experience the disease process for himself but also to develop a real faith in his medicine. His teacher asked him, in effect, if he was willing to trust this medicine with his own life and health. This goes way beyond a merely intellectual commitment or belief. Likewise Dr. Li required some students studying bone-setting to go to a KUNG FU master and have a bone broken on purpose so that they could treat it and experience the treatment from the inside. This kind of training is on a life and death level where all really profound experience takes place. It requires a commitment to one's calling uncommon in western professionals for some time.

Dr. Huang has similarly described how he underwent various fasts and ascetic practices while at the same time practcing QI GONG so that he could literally feel the energy flow in his body. The western history of healing abounds in stories of individuals who through accident have come close to death or who have experienced sensory deprivation, hunger, etc. and who after that found that they experienced subtle levels of reality they had previously not. Eastern disciplines are built on such common experiences. Often they recreate in a controlled way a critical juncture which requires a quantum leap within the student. Such leaps can often not be catalyzed without a certain amount of accepted risk. Such a personal experience of Qi as Dr. Huang's is qualitatively different from an intellectual belief in its existence. Like membership in a famous lineage, such personal experience creates a confidence which can have a pronounced pragmatic effect on the patient. But, if you want to dance to the music, you've got to pay the piper.

Just as not all students are equally intelligent, compassionate, or energetic, so not all students have the same talents. Dr. Li trained Michael in a degree of pulse reading far beyond what is usually encountered today amongst Chinese practitioners. However, the same Dr. Li hardly encouraged another American student to develop pulse-based diagnostic skills at all. Instead he encouraged this student to concentrate on the treatment of BI Syndromes by acupuncture which, in general, does not require extremely sophisticated pulse reading. This emphasizes that each person is different and has different capacities. The creation of standard curricula taught in group classes imposes a rigid, non-responsive, non-flowing and therefore artificial and life-denying structure on a process of human life: growth. Western medicine, as an extension of western culture, has boxed itself into a corner with this approach. Chinese medicine, on the other hand, has favored individual training as a response to the natural impulses of life and it is this life running through its veins that has made its traditionally trained practitioners such effective healers.

However, if the methodology of apprenticeship is so great, why did the few Californians trained by it fare so badly on the state exam mentioned above? The main reason is, in my opinion, because the apprenticeship they underwent was not the same as described in this essay. American preceptorships as established by law in those states which recognize such an educational option are only required to last two or three years. It is assumed that they simply mimic the curricula of schools taught tutorially. Traditional apprenticeships, which should more correctly by termed discipleships, do not last two or three years but often fifteen and a lifetime. The majority of apprenticeships offered in the United States are poor comparisons to the type of teaching I am talking about.

By and large, Americans lack the cultural context to undergo such a training. We stress quick results and time-efficiency. We value facts and external credentials. We believe in independence and doing our own thing. Ted Kaptchuk has said publically that the entire concept of mastership has been and ought to be obsolete in the West since the French Revolution. Traditional Oriental teachers, according to Huang Pao-chin, feel that westerners lack self-control to the point that we are incapable of the real discipline that is part of discipleship. In addition, our economic environment militates against the implementation of this kind of apprenticeship in the United States. It is rare that an American practitioner would have the room and income to support a student studying and interning as an apprentice. In general, American students take up the study of Chinese medicine as adults when they are no longer supported by their parents and may even be supporting a family of their own. Therefore, most Americans' Chinese medical education is part time and not even as extensive or complete as that of TCM school in the PRC.

Given the above, is such a traditional model of education a dinosaur destined to disappear? Although the times are moving in a different direction, I believe it is important to keep alive the vision of this educational option. Most of our problems in this day and age, both health and societal, are due to our seeking quick fixes. We suffer from Time Disease which leads us into a maze of superficiality. It is my opinion that only a profound medicine based on the "perennial philosophy" of mystical insight can redress this Evil Speed at its root. Even if we can implement this type of education rarely, still its presence in our consciousness helps us not to take too seriously and believe too fervently in the inevitability and supremacy of our contemporary system. Certain KUNG FU masters teach Chinese medicine this way here in America and in Taiwan, Hong Kong, and Singapore. There are a couple of schools, such as the Five Branches Institute and the Kotatama Institute, whch try to train the entire person as well as fulfilling state educational requirements. Americans such as Michael Broffman have been trained in this other mode of Chinese medical education and have been recognized by their American peers as possesing a special insight into our art. And Michael has his disciple sweeping the floor of his clinic.

The Chinese have a story about a dragon painted on the wall of a temple. One day, the Emperor, travelling about the realm in disguise, came upon this temple and asked the locals why the dragon had no eyes. They answered that if the dragon were given eyes it would fly up into the sky and no longer perform his duties to the village. The Emperor summoned a painter and ordered the artist to paint in the eyes. As soon as the painter was finished, the dragon began to move and ascended into the heavens. In Chinese, the saying, "Paint dragon (and) dot the eyes" (HUA LONG DIAN JING) means to bring something to its final completion, whereupon it comes alive. This saying is particularly used by Huang Pao-chin to question if one has really understood the heart of a problem or teaching in a living, experiential way. As he says, it took a long time to paint the dragon with all its many scales, but only a second or two to paint in its eyes. Without a doubt, the important thing is the flash of insight which makes a system come alive. In America we all are interested in giving the dragon of Chinese medicine eyes. However, we should not forget that first the picture must be painted scale by scale.

ENDNOTES

1 Manfred Porkert, in "The Intellectual and Social Impulses Behind the Evolution of Traditional Chinese Medicine", appearing in ASIAN MEDICAL SYSTEMS: A COMPARATIVE STUDY, ed. by Charles Leslie, U of CA Press, Berkeley, 1976, states that "up to the 6th century A.D. all traditions were transmitted from master to disciple, and the only way to become a doctor was to apprentice oneself to a practicing physician." Porkert goes on to say:" Then under the Tang, first attempts were made to set up a regular medical school at the capital. From the Sung period, the Great Medical Office (Tai I Chin) became a permanent institution....Most of the graduates of the Medical Office stayed on in the capital, to be delegated only temporarily to the provinces." Drawing a conclusion to his recapitulation of the institution of formal medical schools in China, it is Porkert's opinion that its institutionalization in the Tang and Sung set the stage for its eventual stagnation and decay in the Yuan, Ming, and Qing. "And to all evidence traditional Chinese medicine...has to this day not recovered from the methodological sterilization it suffered as a consequence to its marriage with Confuscianism", i.e. the institutionalized ruling hierarchy. p.70.

2 Ralph Crozier, in "The Ideology of Revivalism in China" appearing in ASIAN MEDICAL SYSTEMS: A COMPARATIVE STUDY, op. cit. states that Chinese medicine's "erosion of its theoretical basis, in an attempt to rationalize and systematize it for standardized teaching ... threaten(s) to dissolve the theoretical basis of Chinese medicine and leave an assortment of remedies and procedures that might be of considerable adaptive value in providing public health care, but would hardly constitute an integral medical system." p. 351.

3 I recently received an invitation to a seminar in Florida on TCM. The title of the seminar was something like "The Proper Diagnosis and Correct Erection of Treatment Plans According to Traditional Chinese Medicine". Although there is a valid distinction between an accurate and inaccurate diagnosis, the contemporary Chinese tendency to insist that there is a "correct" diagnosis and a "correct" treatment suggests a blurring of the conceptual distinction between map and terrain. This stressing of rectitude is characteristically Chinese but has been aggravated by the current authoritarian regime. It echoes mainland Chinese' preoccupation and ultimately paranoia about hewing to the correct party line. This attitude is not meritorious nor is it appropriate that we adopt it here.

4 In my experience, otitis media and tonsilitis in infants and children have a tendency to become chronic if treated by antibiotics. Similarly, vaginitis, cystitis, and PID often become chronic in adults treated antibiotically.

5 See THE LIFE OF MILAREPA, Lhalungpa, Lobsang, trans., E.P. Dutton, NY, 1977, or WOMEN OF WISDOM, Allione, Tsultrim, Routledge & Kegan Paul, London, Boston, etc., 1984 for exemplary biographies.

6 Porkert in op. cit. p. 69 mentions that "the similarity of style and terminology between Taoist and medical texts is no accident, nor is the fact that

many of the early compilers of medical classics were even better known as Taoist adepts -- e.g. Huang Fu-mi, Ko Hung, Tao Hung-chin , and Sun Szu-mo."

[7] Ge Hung, ALCHEMY, MEDICINE, AND RELIGION IN CHINA OF AD 320 (PAO PU TZE NEI PIEN), trans. by James R. Ware, MIT Press, Cambridge & London, 1966, p.212

[8] Ibid. p. 212-13

[9] Rechung Rinpoche, TIBETAN MEDICINE, U of CA Press, Berkeley & LA, 1973, p. 91

[10] Chaitow, Leon, THE ACUPUNCTURE TREATMENT OF PAIN, Thorsons Publishers, UK, 1983, quoted in the AJA, Vol 13, #4, Dec. 1985, p. 400

[11] THE PACIFIC JOURNAL OF ORIENTAL MEDICINE, San Francisco College of Acupuncture & Oriental Medicine, SF, Vol. 2, #2, Summer 1985, p. 60

[12] Tatz, Mark, BUDDHISM & HEALING, University Press of America, Lanham & NY, 1985, p. 95

[13] Clifford, Terry, TIBETAN BUDDHIST MEDICINE & PSYCHIATRY, Samuel Weiser Inc., York Beach, ME, 1984 p. 81

[14] Kaptchuk, Ted, remarks made during a seminar in Denver, Summer 1984

[15] These accounts were given by Michael Broffman in a seminar he taught on theory and practice of Chinese medicine at the Third Annual Rocky Mountain Healing Arts Festival held in August, 1979 outside Boulder, CO, which I attended.

CROSSING POINTS IN TIME

A Discussion of the Use of LUO Points

Contemporary TCM (Traditional Chinese Medicine) acupuncture pays scant attention to the transfer of energy by manipulating the so-called Antique points according to Five Element theory. TCM acupuncture is an "herbalized"[1] version of this art which has gained ascendency in China during this century. This system uses the differentiation of named patterns of disharmony as both the basis of its diagnosis and treatment. Damp Spleen, Flaring of Deficiency Fire of the Heart, Arrogant Liver Yang, and Stagnant Blood in the Blood Chamber are examples of standard TCM patterns of disharmony. Such patterns are diagnosed by comparing three basic groups of criteria: 1) general signs and symptoms, 2) tongue signs, and 3) pulse signs. According to Michael Broffman, tongue diagnosis traditionally was developed by practitioners of NEI KE, Internal herbal medicine.[2] The pulse diagnosis employed by this style is based on that of Li Shi-zhen, the famous Ming dynasty herbalist. Twentieth century practitioners of TCM such as Wang Le-ting have consciously and deliberately created acupuncture protocols based on famous herbal prescriptions where each point or group of points mimics the action of a specific herbal ingredient. Since many American acupuncture schools have adopted this version of acupuncture as the basis for their curriculum this style has also gained ascendency in America today.

However there is another, older style of acupuncture based on the NEI JING, NAN JING, and JIA YI JING rather than on the NEI KE texts of the Jin, Yuan, and Ming dynasties. This older style of acupuncture concerns itself with rebalancing the Qi which flows in the various channels and collaterals as opposed to directly affecting the metabolism of the internal organs. It utilizes all twelve major meridians equally without unduly emphasizing the Yin channels as herbalized TCM acupuncture tends to do. Its diagnosis is primarily based on Wang Shu-he's pulse theory of the late Han dynasty. Its methodology for altering the flow of Qi through the channels and collaterals is primarily by manipulating the Antique points according to Five Element and Ten Stems theories. This style of acupuncture has been preserved in Japan to this day. It is also widely practiced in Europe, due largely to the influence of the Vietnamese Nguyen

Van Nghi. Unfortunately its English language proponents both in America and elsewhere have suffered from shoddy scholarship concerning the historicity of their tradition and because of this have come under heavy criticism from their TCM counterparts. This, parenthetically, has created a schism in the American acupuncture community which has had and continues to have a negative effect on the profession.

Although I am a practitioner of TCM and have studied TCM acupuncture at the Shanghai College of Traditional Chinese Medicine, it is my opinion that TCM acupuncture is a tour de force. Acupuncture and herbal therapy are essentially different methods for re-establishing homeostasis in the human bodymind. Post Song scholars, trying to create a single orthodox theory of treatment, have tried to homogenize the theories of the NEI JING and the SHANG HAN LUN. However, Chinese herbalism was not created by the same individuals who created acupuncture and there are a number of fundamental differences between the two. It is my belief that acupuncture's pre-eminent value is in re-establishing the free, regular, and balanced flow of energy through the network of channels and collaterals. It seems to me that even contemporary Chinese TCM practitioners recognize this fact since acupuncture is largely relegated to the treatment of musculo-skeletal, i.e. meridian, problems in Chinese clinics. To employ acupuncture as if it mimicked herbal therapy and to base acupuncture treatment on herbal methods of diagnosis I believe misses the point of acupuncture and squanders its potential.

As a practitioner of TCM, I have long held the belief that a comprehensive treatment plan utilizing both acupuncture and herbs should not simply duplicate itself using both modalities. Rather it is my opinion that the clinician should determine, based on theory, experience, and in a conscious and rational way, what aspects of a patient's condition should be treated by each and when. Therefore I believe it is possible to practice TCM herbalism and simultaneously practice "energy transfer" acupuncture not based on a TCM BIAN ZHENG but rather on the immediate balance of energy within the channels and collaterals as assessed by the pulse. However, there are few contemporary practitioners in the US capable of transmitting this art. The unscholarly and uncritical approach taken by the Worsley school, the main proponents of energy transfer or so-called Five Element acupuncture in America, casts a pall of suspicion over their entire approach. That leaves primarily Japanese proponents of this style, and, due to the long and deep animosities between the Chinese and Japanese, I see little realistic co-operation between these two nationalities at American acupuncture schools within this generation. One only has to observe the rivalry and division between Chinese and Japanese style practitioners in New Mexico to lose hope in such a direct means of cross-pollenization.

That means that American TCM acupuncturists who question the supremacy of their style and who wish to deepen their understanding must largely depend upon the written and translated literature. However, this very quickly becomes confusing since there is a welter of conflicting opinion upon the correct methodology for balancing the energy in the meridians utilizing Five Element theory and the Antique points. Leaving aside the obvious discrepancy between simple Five Element and Ten Stems theories, this confusion is well exemplified by the various opinions concerning the use of the Luo Connecting points.

In English TCM acupuncture literature little is said about the nature and use of the Luo points. ESSENTIALS OF CHINESE ACUPUNCTURE says the Luo points may be used to treat two Externally-Internally (BIAO LI) related channels and also disease in the area supplied by two such channels. Externally-Internally related channels refers to the pairing of Yin and Yang meridians. For instance, the Hand Yang Ming Large Intestine channel is the External member of the Yin Yang pair of which the Hand Tai Yin Lung channel is the Internal member. ACUPUNCTURE: A COMPREHENSIVE TEXT simply adds that when symptomology effects two such paired meridians, the Luo point of the meridian on which the majority of symptoms appear can be needled effectively.

ACUPUNCTURE ENERGY IN HEALTH AND DISEASE states that there are two separate pathways which originate at the Luo points. One is the Luo Connecting channel mentioned above. The other is the so-called Longitudinal Luo which to some extent parallels the main channel and extend the channel's influence to areas adjacent to its main course.[3] This discussion of the use of the Luo points will confine itself, however, to accessing the Luo Connecting channel only. The pathways of the Longitudinal Luo and their application in clinical practice is likewise an area of debate and confusion but I think it is safe to say that they do not play a significant part in energy transfer acupuncture vis a vis the Five Elements.

While all sources agree that the Luo Connecting channels connect the paired Yin Yang main meridians, there is no universal agreement on how they connect. Felix Mann in ACUPUNCTURE: THE ANCIENT CHINESE ART OF HEALING AND HOW IT WORKS SCIENTIFICALLY shows one Connecting channel running from the Luo point of a Yang Meridian to the Luo point of its paired Yin meridian. For instance, LIE QUE (Lu 7), the Luo point of the Hand Tai Yin, is connected to PIAN LI (LI 6), the Luo point of the Hand Yang Ming and vice versa.[4] Based on this assumption Mann gives the following guidelines for manipulating the Qi through the Luo points: If one or another of a paired Yin Yang set of meridians is Excess or Deficient, one can tonify the Luo point of the Deficient meridian or disperse the Luo point of the Excess meridian. The implication is that energy will be drawn from the paired opposite meridian to tonify the Deficiency and that energy will be dispersed to the opposite meridian to reduce Excess. Although Mann does not state it explicitly, the logical inference is that Qi can potentially flow in both directions across this single Connecting channel.

Mann gives two other uses of the Luo points not found elsewhere in the English literature. He states that the Luo points can be used to equalize the bilateral courses of a single meridian if these are found to be out of balance, presumably through Akabane testing or some other such method. In other words, if the right side of the Hand Tai Yin is Excess vis a vis the left side, one can disperse right LIE QUE. Whereas, if the right Hand Tai Yin is Deficient vis a vis the left, right LIE QUE can be tonified. In addition Mann says that the Luo points can also restore balance between the meridians on which they are found and the meridian related to them by the Midday-Midnight law. For instance, the Hand Tai Yin is at high tide diurnally from three to five AM; while the Foot Tai Yang is at high tide from three to five PM. Therefore, from three to five AM when the Hand Tai Yin is at high tide, the Foot Tai Yang is simultaneously at low tide. If the Hand Tai Yin is Excess, dispersal of its Luo point will tonify any Deficiency of the Foot Tai Yang and vice versa.

Two contemporary Chinese sources from Taiwan, where Japanese influence on

ANATOMY OF CONNECTING LUO ACCORDING TO WOOLERTON & MCLEAN

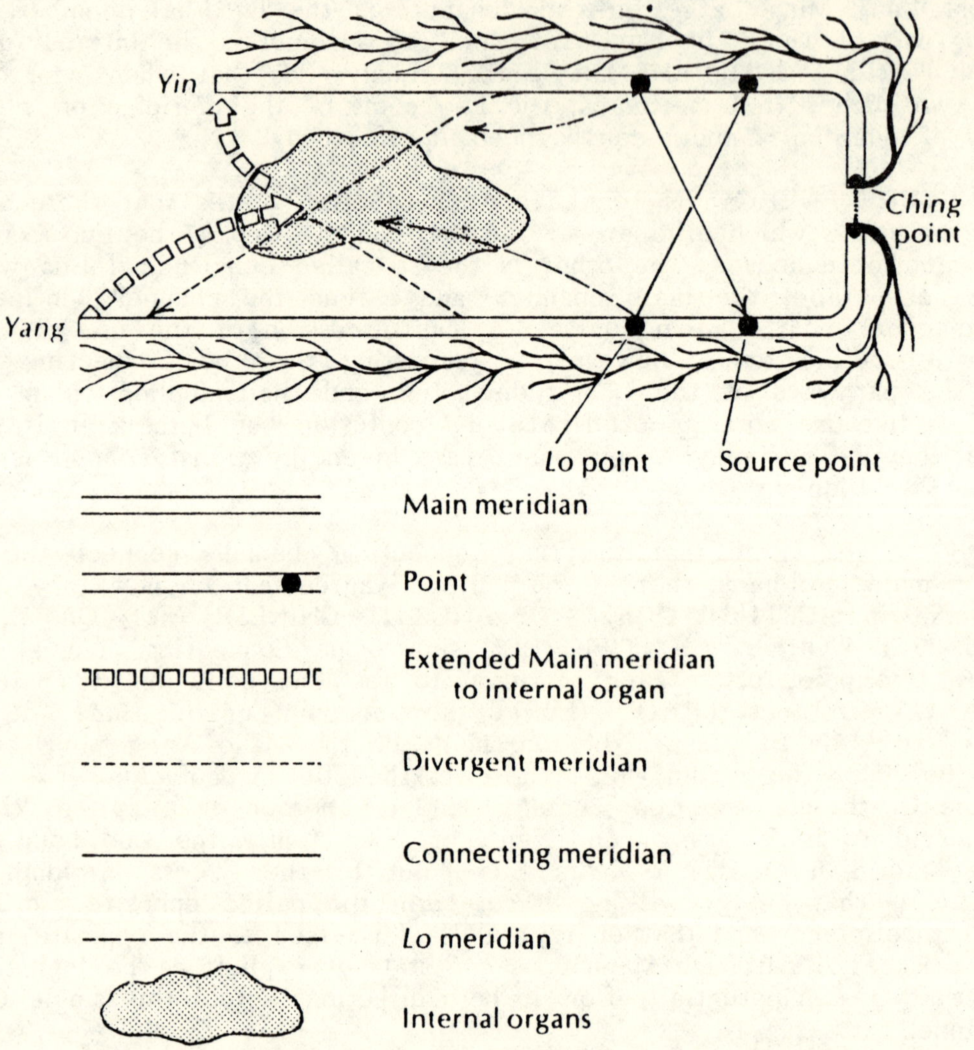

ANATOMY OF CONNECTING LUO ACCORDING TO FELIX MANN

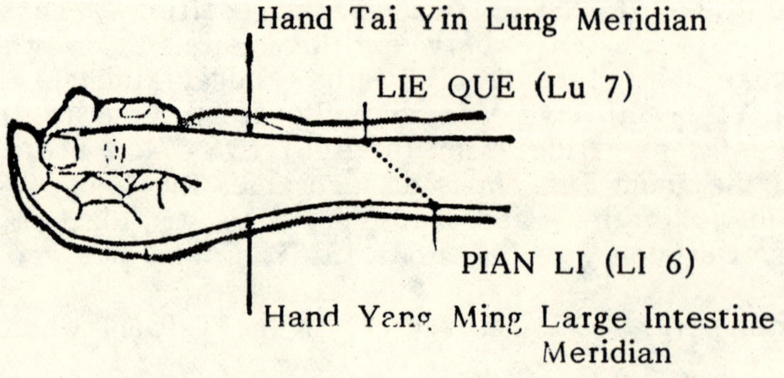

the practice of Chinese medicine has been pervasive since the turn of the century, disagree with Mann concerning the implied two way flow of the Luo Connecting channels. Wu Wei-ping says that energy flows to the meridian on which the Luo point is found.[5] Wu states that if the Foot Jue Yin is Excess and the Foot Tai Yin is Deficient one must needle the Wood point on the Foot Tai Yin, i.e. Yin Bai (Sp 1) and the Luo point of the Foot Shao Yang, GUANG MING (GB 37). The Excess in the Foot Jue Yin will then flow to the Foot Shao Yang and thence to the Foot Tai Yin. The transfer from Foot Shao Yang to Foot Tai Yin is effected through the KE cycle according to Ten Stems theory. Tao Hsi-yu, on the other hand, has stated explicitly in lectures here in America that the Qi only flows from the merdian on which the Luo point is found. Therefore, to effect this same transfer cited above he says one must needle LI GOU (Liv 5), not GUANG MING. However, Dr. Tao does not use Ten Stems theory and for him needling YIN BAI would have been sufficient in the case above. In any case, Dr. Tao says that it is very important to be aware of the direction of flow of the Luo and to choose the appropriate Luo point, i.e. the point which opens the Luo to the coupled meridian.

According to ACUPUNCTURE ENERGY IN HEALTH AND DISEASE and the Occidental Institute of Chinese Studies' course on Modern and Traditional Acupuncture, Qi flows from the Luo on the meridian on which it is found to the Yuan Source point on the coupled opposite meridian. OICS bases its information largely on the work of Nguyen Van Nghi, the Vietnamese Grandmaster of European acupuncture. The authors of the OICS course material state: "the (Yuan) point receives and absorbs the energy coming from the opposed coupled meridian and this is why the NEI JING insists on the character 'of absorption' of this point."[6] OICS gives a number of examples of protocols for effecting the transfer of energy across the Luo Conecting channel. Basically they recommend needling both the Luo point on the one merdian and the Yuan Source point on the coupled meridian. Depending upon whether one tonfies or disperses these points the energy will flow in either direction. For instance, if the Hand Tai Yin is Excess and the Hand Yang Ming is Deficient, one can tonify HE GU (LI 4) and disperse LIE QUE. Tonification of LIE QUE and dispersion of HE GU would have just the opposite effect.

OICS goes on to say that the Luo points only regulate imbalances caused by Internal disequilibrium. One should never use the Luo/Yuan combination when treating an External disease thus allowing entry to the deeper energetic layers to the pathogen. Although this is a logical consideration, I am reminded of the well-known TCM protocol for Wind Cold Invasion of the Lung which employs LIE QUE, HE GU, FENG MEN (Bl 12), and FENG CHI (GB 20) and which is often remarkably effective.

TCM has largely abandoned Five Element energy transfer acupuncture because there is so much disagreement over just this kind of theoretical point. In the dichotomy between Rational and Empirical medicine posited by Coulter[7], energy transfer acupuncture is a rational system based on theoretical principles. TCM acupuncture, on the other hand, tends to rely on empirically proven combinations. When these combinations can be explained by ancient principles, so much the better, but even if they cannot, their effectiveness is what counts. If a number of different schools each posit contradictory theories and principles regarding the use of such a potentially important group of points as the Luo points and all equally claim that their methods work, can any one of these theories really be true? The tendency in contemporary TCM is to say that all this theorizing is GUO FEN, i.e. too much or beyond belief, that simply needling the point is enough to effect homeostasis between the coupled meridians without regard to direction of flow or BU FA or XIE FA (tonification and dispersion techniques).

That may be satisfying to many clinicians who are simply interested in dealing with a patient's immediate symptoms and who do not have the time and interest to ponder the long-term effects of their treatments. That may also satisfy those who are unaware that remarkable cures with only a couple of needles and a couple of treatments have been effected by historical Chinese and contemporary Japanese, European, and American practitioners of energy transfer acupuncture. Dr. Tao learned acupuncture from his uncle as a teenager in pre-World War II Peking. After the war he lived and practiced in Taiwan for thirty years. Dr. Tao uses energy transfer acupuncture based on Wang Shu-he's pulse diagnosis employing mainly the sixty-six Antique points and the Luo and Yuan points. I have seen him cure patients with only one or two needles in one or two sessions whom I had treated unsuccessfully with TCM BIAN ZHENG acupuncture over a protracted period of time. Kiko Matsumoto in FIVE ELEMENTS AND TEN STEMS describes some of the Five Element acupuncture cures of MSSRS. Yanagiya, Okabe, Inoue, Honma, and Shudo.[8] Wu Wei-ping states that due to the profound reflection on the Five Elemental relationship of the Antique points "the ancient Masters of Acupuncture could cure within a few minutes and with but one or two needles."[9]

For me the answer to the conundrum of how all these opposing theories and contradictory techniques can achieve pragmatically good results is based on the metaphysical nature of Qi and the traditional Oriental method of training. Traditionally, acupuncture was taught in a Master-disciple relationship. This training included rules of behavior which were designed to instil absolute confidence in the methods and opinions of the Master. Often, as with Dr. Tao, one's Master was selected based upon family relationship, not on a comparison of merits. Even when the relationship was entered into after having compared the teachings and techniques of several potential Masters, once the bond of discipleship was forged a large number of social and even religious factors were employed to create faith and trust in the particular system in which one was being trained. Because, from the Buddhist, Taoist, and Neo-Confuscianist points of view, Qi and Mind are essentially identical, the state of mind of the practitioner is vital in effecting the appropriate response to treatment. In Qigong it is said that the Mind leads the Qi. Qigong players lead the Qi to a body part or organ by visualizing or imagining that it is indeed going there. I believe that what happens when a needle is inserted into a patient by an acupuncturist is largely dependent upon the strength of belief of both the patient <u>and</u> the practitioner. Ted Kaptchuk was once discussing the use of TIAN FU (Lu 3) with a Worsleyan practitioner. The Worsleyan was horrified that Kaptchuk talked of using this point very early on in a course of treatments. The Worsleyan expected and experienced extreme cathartic responses in patients on which this point is needled. Kaptchuk replied that obviously the Worsleyan endowed his acupuncture with much more power than he himself did. If such is true, then doubt may be one of the most important factors in the success or failure of a given treatment. As described above, a large part of the training of a traditonal acupuncturist was aimed at eradicating doubt.

In our modern Age of Information we assume that the more different ideas we are exposed to the closer we come to the Truth. That is true only if we can pierce through the welter of confusing ideas to grasp the essential truth or meaning behind the apparent contradictions. The greatest faith is based on understanding. However, if we fail, out of intellectual and emotional laziness, to dig deeply for the truth, we will be tossed this way and that upon the winds of superficiality. Without the single-mindedness which comes with conviction, little of import can be accomplished.

Huang Shu-li, a Chinese doctor now living in Taiwan, explained to his apprentice, Donn Hayes, that there are three stages in the development of an acupuncturist. In the first stage the student mimics by rote and unerringly all their teacher's methods and instructions. In the second stage the student begins to question some of the reasons behind the teacher's instructions and begins to experiment on his or her own. In the third stage the student arrives at their own understanding. This is the stage where the student matures into their own right. Dr. Huang said that because of the single-minded faith in the first stage the practitioner's results will be good although limited. In the second stage the practitioner's results will actually diminish due to lack of conviction and a wavering mind/Qi. If the student makes it to the third stage, their results will again improve, in fact surpassing those of the first stage, since the singleness of mind created by mature understanding is superior to blind, unreasonning faith.

We cannot turn back the hands of time. As a profession in America it seems to me we have entered the second of Dr. Huang's stages, in many cases having skipped the first. Picking a system and adhering to it by closing our eyes to all other possibilities does not work for most of us Americans, nor is that a mature approach. Having bitten the apple of knowledge, we must go through the ordeal of transcending that knowledge. We cannot and should not pretend a primitive naiveté. For me that means consciously acknowledging the role Mind plays behind technique and developing conviction in the power of intention. As long as we continue to focus the power of our intent through the form of inserting needles, we must, by necessity, choose to employ certain techniques. These techniques may vary from individual to individual within certain limitations. For instance, all sources agree, both classical and contemporary, that the Luo points connect in some way the Qi of two paired meridians. What is important, however, is that the practitioner believes in their technique and achieves good pragmatic, clinical results in their patients, not that its validity be proven by some supposedly objective test. As Bishop Berkeley and the Yogacarya Buddhist philosophers have both asserted, in fact there is no such thing as a provable external or objective reality. All proofs of such a reality are experienced subjectively by the mind. Therefore the Mind is all we know and can ever know as we ceaselessly traverse the changing strands of time.

ENDNOTES

1 Kaptchuk, Ted, "Acupuncture in the West -- a discussion between Ted Kaptchuk, Giovanni Maciocia, Felicity Moir, and Peter Deadman", THE JOURNAL OF CHINESE MEDICINE, UK, No. 17, Jan. 1985, p. 26

2 Broffman, Michael, lecture at the 3rd Annual Rocky Mtn. Healing Arts Festival, Colorado, August 1979

3 Woolerton. H.& McLean,C.J., ACUPUNCTURE ENERGY IN HEALTH & DISEASE Thorsons Publishers Ltd., UK, 1979, p. 38

4 Mann, Felix, ACUPUNCTURE: THE ANCIENT CHINESE ART OF HEALING AND HOW IT WORKS SCIENTIFICALLY, Vintage Books, NYC, 1973, p. 122

5 Wu Wei-ping, xeroxed pages given to me by Daniel Santos of New Mexico from a book by this author which is out of print, a copy of which I have not been able to find. p. 165-166

6 OICS, Modern & Traditional Acupuncture, an introductory course, Lesson 26, p. 7

7 Coulter, H.L., DIVIDED LEGACY: A HISTORY OF THE SCHISM IN MEDICAL THOUGHT, Weehawken Book Co., Wash., DC, 1975

8 Matsumoto, Kiko & Birch, Stephen, FIVE ELEMENTS AND TEN STEMS, Paradigm Publications, Higganum, CT, 1983(?), p. 169-189

9 Wu Wei-ping, op. cit., p. 166